The Case against

Sugar

Your guide to quitting Sugar and Breakfast and Baby Recipes with Zero or Low Sugar Content

Stacy Kennedy

ISBN-13: 978-1543173123

ISBN-10: 1543173128

.

Table of Contents

Introduction

In April 2013, I decided to finally do without sugar. After a ten-weeks start-up program, I found life without the white crumbs getting better and my body feeling lighter (including my own - six pounds less on the ribs and a much better skin tone), so I decided to stick with it. Towards the end of the year I had it a little pretty touch - Christmas cookies and those wine were too tempting! - but 2014 was a sugar-free comeback! Big time!

Since then I have taken time to understand nutrition and diet as it relates to healthy living. My goal with this book and the subsequent sugar free cookbooks that I am writing is to give you all the information in one place, so that you will not have to struggle when you are ready to live sugar free.

Like I wrote earlier, I will be releasing short special and focus sugar free cookbooks soon. Be on the lookout.

Stacy Kennedy.

2017

2. What is sugar?

Whether in chocolate, ice cream, yoghurt, ketchup or ready-to-serve meals - sugar is omnipresent in our lives. Often we do not even know that sugar was one of the main ingredients in our just consumed food. But more about that later.

What is sugar at all? The ordinary household sugar, also known as sucrose, is obtained from sugar cane and sugar beet and consists of glucose (glucose) and fructose (fruit sugar). In addition to conventional household sugar, there are of course other types of sugar, such as fruit sugar, glucose, malt sugar or milk sugar.

Sugar, whether as a food or confectionery, plays a major role in our diet. That was not always so. Even 150 years ago, people took 20 times less sugar than they do today.

Sugar consumption

On average, the people nowadays eat 40 kilos of sugar a year. Of course, honey and the sugar contained in fruits are also included of course. Since sugar is used exclusively for energy but does not contain any healthy nutrients, vitamins or minerals, it is often referred to as "empty energy". Long-chain sugar molecules, so-called multiple sugars, are found in starch-containing foods such as pod fruits or cereals. For the digestion and utilization of multiple sugars, our body needs much longer time compared to single or double sugar, so that a whole grain or a potato dish take much longer to digest than a piece of cake.

It is clear that cancer, diabetes and overweight are inextricably linked to excessive sugar consumption. Therefore, the World Health Organization (WHO) calls for the consumption of sugar to be reduced from currently 100g per day per head to 25g - equivalent to 6 teaspoons of sugar per day.

Attention: Sugar has many names

Admittedly, it is not so easy to limit the consumption of sugar because the number of industrially manufactured products that do not contain sugar is not exactly large. A glance at the list of ingredients can provide clarity in this case. But beware! Because often only the conventional sugars derived from sugar beet or sugar cane must actually be identified as "sugars" or "sucrose" in the list of ingredients.

If, for example, the sugar is replaced by dextrose, lactose, glucose syrup, invert sugar syrup or maltrodextrin, the sugar content in the product is the same. However, the household sugar contained in the product moves further back in the list of ingredients. The consumer, who believes in the supposedly lower sugar content, is misled here. A glance at the carbohydrate content of the product can provide clarity. Here is the small but fine statement "Carbohydrates - of sugar", which gives information about the actual sugar content of the product.

3. How healthy is sugar?

Not without reason, many of us have a bad conscience when eating sweet treats, chocolate and cakes. We know all too well that sugar can lead to obesity, caries and diabetes. But what about the reproaches? How healthy or unhealthy is household sugar really?

Sugar is addictive and bad. But why is that? Interestingly, sugary foods actually have a similar effect on the brain as alcohol or nicotine because the sugar consumption leads to an increased release of dopamine. Dopamine is an important brain messenger for the Brain Reward Center, revealing to the body: "That was good, I want more of it." Similar to the way, the body responds to the consumption of nicotine or alcohol. Anyone who drastically reduces their sugar consumption may have to deal with the symptoms of sugar deprivation. What does these symptoms look like? Sugar deprivation can lead to headache, lack of strength, fatigue, bad mood, but also by the constant craving for sugar.

Is sugar harmful to health?

The fact that the rising consumption of sugar is associated with the increase in obesity, according to nutritionists is obvious. From an evolutionary point of view, the desire for sugar is quite understandable. In ancient times, sweet, ripe fruits corresponded to new energy supply. The energy gained from sugar is, however, no longer required by our bodies today, since carbohydrates from fully-fledged foods provide us with sufficient energy.

The oversupply of sweet and the excess sugar fed by sugars favor obesity. But also skin diseases, caries, diabetes and cardiovascular disease can be attributed to excessive sugar consumption.

Sugar Causes caries?

If we consume sugary foods, a not insignificant part of the sugar will adhere to the teeth. The bacteria on the teeth absorb the sugar, digest it, and excrete the indigestible acids, which ultimately become caries. In contrast to sweeteners and sugar substitutes, which cannot be metabolized by oral fluids and thus do not cause tooth decay, sugar is the most dangerous caries-causing substance.

Does sugar lead to Concentration Weakness?

The glycemic value is used to measure how much the blood glucose level increases after consumption of carbohydrates. If we take sweets or products from extract flasks, the blood glucose level rises, but falls immediately. This has the consequence that the next craving for sugar is not long in coming. The greater the fluctuations of the blood glucose level, the more the desire for sweetness. Fatigue, weakness in concentration, irritability and impaired drive are further consequences of an unstable blood glucose level.

The goal should therefore be to keep the blood glucose level as stable as possible. Whole grain products and vegetables are the best.

Since household sugar is therefore not wrongly criticized to make ill, the question arises of alternatives. Which sweeteners are harmless? What are the advantages and disadvantages of the consumption of honey, Agave juice and Co.? Next I present you ten sweeteners, which are alternatives to cane sugar.

4. Sugar without calories - does it exist?

Every one of us likes to have fun. However, since sugars can lead to obesity and diabetes and, among other things, adversely affect dental health, nutritionists advise to drastically reducing the consumption of sugar. The question is quickly: Is there sugar without calories?

In principle, it can be said that household sugar, regardless of type, contains the same amount of calories, namely, 4.0 kilocalories or 16.8 kJ per gram of sugar. Consequently, 20g of sugar contain literally 80 calories.

What are good alternatives to sugar?

You can rationalize it and try to convince yourself as you want - if you take sugar, you do not do anything good to your body. Also, many health issues such as diabetes or obesity. I am talking about limiting the consumption of sugars and avoiding healthy alternatives to sugars. The following sugar generators are particularly suitable:

- honey
- Bananas
- Dates
- Maple syrup
- Agave syrup
- Coconut nectar
- Stevia

Anyone who thinks about feeding healthily in the future more consciously should not replace his sugar consumption 1: 1 with a sugar substitute but should try to wean his taste buds slowly but surely from sugary food. Because with the regular enjoyment of sweet drinks and food our taste buds dull off. If we suddenly eat less sweet, we often feel the food as bland and tasteless. Therefore, nutritionists advise that the body should be wean step by step from the consumption of sugar. This may take two to three weeks. The result can be seen however: sweet food and beverages are often found after the sugar cessation as too sweet and tasted no more.

What is the effect of sugar on insulin levels?

As stated in the article "What is sugar?", Sugar has a high glyx value. This ensures that the blood glucose level rises faster in the body than in the case of foods such as whole grain products or vegetables with a low Glyx. But in turn - what causes a high blood glucose level caused by the consumption of sugar?

• When the blood glucose level rises, the hormone insulin, which is formed in the pancreas, is poured out. As a rule, there is a linear connection: the higher the blood glucose level, the more insulin is made available. Through this hormone the cells in the human body can now process the energy from sugar, protein or other energy sources and convert it to energy. Especially in small children, one can observe that the activity and energy after the consumption of chocolate and other sugary foods or drinks increases strongly.

• If the insulin value is too high, the human cells process a lot of energy; It comes to a kind of stress of the cell, since the energy exchange is almost exaggerated.

• If there is a constant insulin excess, the processing mechanisms of the cell are disturbed. There is a deficit of the necessary energy for the cells, which leads to the body usually not getting enough energy. At the same time, the energy remains in the blood and is ultimately stored in the fetal cells.

Sugar should therefore be handled very carefully - not only because of its high energy content, but also because of its direct effect on the blood glucose level of the body.

5. Life without sugar - Benefits of a sugar-free diet

The fact that a sugar-free diet significantly reduces the risk of obesity, diabetes, hypertension, gout, osteoporosis and caries is likely to be known to many. However, a sugar-free diet brings additional benefits. If you have been thinking of restricting your consumption of sugar or to feed yourself completely sugar-free, the following facts will surely serve you as a decision-making aid to a sugar-free diet:

1. You feel fitter and healthier

Statistics shows that we eat an average of 40 kilos of sugar a year. There are many who know that sugar is directly related to caries, diabetes, overweight, and cardiovascular disease. The fact that he also leads to immunodeficiency, osteoporosis, digestive complaints, hyperactivity, drive and energy loss as well as to depression, is gladly displaced.

Sugar is strongly acidic. The imbalance of the acid-base balance or the over-acidification of the body means that we feel tired, limp and energy less. Also common colds and headaches can indicate an imbalance in the acid-base budget. A sugar-free diet can help you on the way to a balanced acid-base household.

Not to forget: A balanced, sugar-free diet keeps the blood glucose level constant and sweets or hot starter beaks are a thing of the past.

2. You have more energy

Excessive consumption of sugar makes sluggish and drowsy, as the insulin level rises up and the body pours out insulin and tryptophan. By the insulin, the elimination of fatty acids is prevented and thus the fat burning is blocked. The tryptophan is converted by the body into the happiness hormone serotonin, which leads us to prefer to immediately put a round on the ear.

If, on the other hand, full-fledged, sugar-free and largely unprocessed foods, which provide the body with sufficient antioxidants, vitamins, iron, water and proteins, one will get more energetic through the day.

3. You increase your concentration

Research shows that the consumption of sugar can lead to concentration difficulties. Especially children react very energetically, sometimes almost hyperactively to the consumption of sugar. The reason is that the sugar drives the energy to peak values, but then the blood glucose lowers quickly to the necessary level. The performance curve of the child therefore accelerates upwards in the short term, but sinks just as quickly, so that the sugar can lead to subsequent fatigue and weaknesses in concentration.

4. You look younger and better

Sugar not only deprives the body of important minerals and vitamins, but also has a negative impact on the external appearance. In the chemical process known as glycation, sugar molecules adhere to collagen fibers, which ultimately lose their suppleness. The skin loses its flexibility and can no longer counteract wrinkles.

5. You hold your weight or lose a few pounds

A medium- and long-term weight reduction can be associated with a reduction in sugar content. Obesity and obesity lead to a lower life expectancy, but also increase the risk of diabetes, cancer or osteoarthritis.

According to a study by the Monash University in Melbourne, sugar causes the cells responsible for brain control for appetite control to die. The consequence: a stronger hunger feeling and ultimately obesity.

6. You have healthier teeth

Tooth caries is produced by converting the sugar in the diet into lactic acid, which attacks the molten tooth. The sweeteners look different, since these cannot be converted to acid by the bacteria in the mouth. Here, in particular, xylitol is to be emphasized, which even contributes to dental health. For drinks without sugar, however, it is worth taking a look at the list of ingredients. The maltodextrin, a sugar substitute which is not a conventional household sugar, can be found here, however, just as sugar caries can cause caries.

6. Fructose - is there no sugar in it?

Fructose belongs to the group of carbohydrates and is regarded by many as a healthy alternative to sugar. Fruit is found in nature, for example, in fruit and honey. For example, the proportion of fructose in grapes or bananas is up to 50%, in cherries and apples up to 60%. The top runners are raisins and dry fruits. For example, little fructose contains fruits such as papayas, berries or citrus fruits.

Since fructose is usually associated with healthy vegetables, fructose is commonly considered healthy. However, as the name suggests, it is a normal sugar, such as glucose. Fructose is also present in bound form in conventional household sugar, since sucrose is a two-sugar sugar consisting of glucose and fructose.

However, fructose does not occur only in fruits. Especially in the USA, fructose is highly concentrated as "High Fructose Corn Syrup" in ready-to-eat meals and soft drinks. If you are interested in avoiding fructose, you should bear in mind that there is no obligatory labeling requirement for fruit sugar. Therefore, fructose can also hide behind the following terms: fruit juices, corn syrup, juice concentrate, corn sugar, invert sugar syrup, fruit extract, glucose fructose syrup.

Fructose, i.e., fruit sugar, is often chosen as a sweet alternative to sugar.

Advantages of fructose

• Fructose is 1.14 times sweeter than sugar. This means that less fruit is needed to achieve the same sweetness as sugar.

- Fructose is metabolized without insulin. The glycemic index of fructose is 20, which means that fructose increases slowly the blood glucose level.

Disadvantages of fructose

- The body tolerates fructose. However, there are also people (about 20% of the population) who are suffering from the so-called fructose malabsorption, so they cannot metabolize fructose, and therefore they can only eat it to a very limited extent. Otherwise, cramps, flatulence and diarrhea are the result.

- Fructose has often been used for diabetic foods, as it is metabolized without insulin. However, according to various studies, the use of fructose in food is not useful since the increased consumption of fructose can lead to an overweight.

• The German Institute for Nutrition Research also published a study in 2005 that showed that the uptake of fructose significantly increased the body fat absorption of mice. Following the study, it was shown that fructose leads to higher increase in human fat than glucose. In addition, the storage of fats is increased by the consumption of fruit sugar.

• Since fructose is almost consume completely in the liver, fruit sugar can not only lead to increased uric acid formation but also to a fatty liver.

• Not to mention that fructose sounds like something natural, healthy. This often leads to an uncontrolled consumption of sweetened foods.

To conclude, fructose is not necessarily the healthier alternative to sugar. Especially as fruit sugar provides 4 kilocalories per gram - as much as conventional household sugar. Nevertheless, one should not completely avoid fructose. Rather, it is important to enjoy fruit juices in moderation - preferably in the form of fresh fruits and vegetables. This provides our body, in addition to fructose, a lot of nutrients and dietary fibers. However, the proportion of vegetables in any case should be above the proportion of fruit.

7. Do you suffer from fructose intolerance?

If the consumption of fruit regularly leads to stomach cramps and flatulence, there may be a fructose intolerance behind. All about the symptoms and what you can do about it

What exactly is a fructose intolerance?

Fructose intolerance * (also called fructosemal absorption) is a food intolerance and not an allergy, as is often the case. Fructose (better known as fruit sugar) cannot be properly digested due to a lack of protein in the body. The reason being that fructose is normally transported to the blood through the intestinal mucosa, but a portion of the necessary transport system is not available in sufficient quantity, which means that the fruit sugar cannot be absorbed completely. This then move to the colon, where it is decomposed bacterially. The resulting gases and acids ensure, among other things, unpleasant flatulence, abdominal cramps and abdominal cramps.

Do you suffer from a fructose intolerance?

Whether you are suffering from a fructose intolerance, you first of all recognize the typical symptoms: In addition to flatulence and stomach pain, diarrhea, nausea, bloating and even headache are also common. The complaints usually only occur 30 minutes to 2 hours later, after the food of fructose - containing food.

Many sufferers also develop a kind of natural protection by instinctively avoiding anything sweet and having no desire for sugar at all. Anyone who often feels tired and chipped, or is often sick, may also suffer from a fructose intolerance. "A reliable diagnosis can only be given by a doctor, however, an intolerance is not always present behind the complaints, because an" overdose "fruit sugar cannot be easily digested without any problem". However, anyone who already reacts to smaller amounts of juice or fruit, honey or jam with diarrhea, flatulence and co.

How to diagnose fructose intolerance?

The diagnosis is usually performed with the aid of a special breath test, in which the physician measures the hydrogen content in the respiratory air. Why? As already mentioned, caused by the bacterial degradation of the fructose in the intestinal gases - including hydrogen - which can be detected in the exhaled air. The principle of the test: Measure the hydrogen content once on a sober stomach and then drink a fructose solution, then repeat the measurement every 30 minutes and observe whether or in what speed and intensity the hydrogen content increases It can then be concluded whether a fructose intolerance exists. " Since several measurements are taken successively, the examination takes about 3 hours. You can before the test itself, detect which foods may be suspicious or cause discomfort.

Diagnosis:Fructose intolerance. What now?

No fear, even with the diagnosis Fructose intolerance one can eat healthy and balanced and above all also enjoy. Fructose intolerance can neither be medically treated nor cured, but with an adapted, fructose- poor diet, one can live as far as possible without complaint. The goal should be to change your diet in the long term and completely.

At the beginning is the waiting period. In this first phase, fructose should be avoided as far as possible. Especially sweet drinks such as sodas, cola and fruit juice drinks as well as artificially enriched with fruit sugar or the more popular glucose fructose syrup (corn syrup) are to be avoided. Afterwards you start to test individual foods to find out how much fruit you can tolerate individually. For those who know their Fructose-Limit can live quite normal despite their "handicap", this book can help you master the first, unaccustomed time of the changeover with the help of tasty recipes and tips.

What foods are allowed in a fructose intolerance?

The following foods are usually tolerated without problems:

- Cereal products
- Dairy products (without fruit)
- Vegetables such as asparagus, lettuce, chicory, spinach, leaf salads, avocados
- Potatoes
- Fish, meat, poultry, eggs

Fruits are often problematic, at least in the beginning. However, some varieties such as rhubarb or prickly pears are relatively low in fructose and are therefore often well tolerated. Absolute No Go are dry fruits, fruit juices, jam and honey, because here hides a lot of fructose. You should also keep your fingers from wine, sparkling wine, beer and fruit teas. All dos and don'ts with a fructose-poor diet, by the way, you will find at the end of this chapter in an overview table.

Is it impossible to eat fruit in a fructose intolerance?

Anyone who thinks he has to remove fruit completely from his menu, can convince the expert: "Nobody should give up fresh fruit and vegetables altogether because these foods are our main supplier of vitamins and minerals." It is important to know what fruits you are taking, Because the right fructose-glucose ratio is important here: since grape-sugar favors the utilization of fruit sugar, fruit varieties with high dextrose and low sugar content such as honey melons, bananas or papaya are often well tolerated Apples, pears, cherries, plums, mangoes, watermelons, kiwis and grapes.

For those who do not want to do without cherries and watermelons in the summer, for example, here is a tip for you "Sprinkle a teaspoon of dextrose (glucose) over the fruit, making the fruits (with the prudence to be enjoyed) more palatable."

Caution for sugar substitutes

Also pay attention to the ingredients list of products, because not only fructose but also sugar substitutes should be avoided. These include:

- Sorbitol or sorbitol (E420)
- Isomalt / isomaltitol (E 953)
- Lactitol / lactitol (E 966)
- Maltitol / maltitol (E 965)
- Mannitol / mannitol (E 421)
- Xylitol / xylitol (E967)

What can I do with a slip?

"Only the hot water bottle helps," says the nutritionist. A toilet within range should also always be in such a case. "As soon as the villain has left, you will soon get better."

All do's and don'ts a fructose-poor diet

Critical (usually incompatible with fructose intolerance)	Harmless (usually tolerated with fructose intolerance)
(E 423), maltitol (E 965), polysaccharides / oligosaccharides (in large quantities), sugar substitutes, sugar substitutes, sugar substitutes,	Glucose / dextrose = glucose lactose = milk sugar Maltose = malt sugar
Honey, jam, cornflakes, corn, soy, oat flakes, peanuts	
Mayonnaise, ketchup	
Finished products such as fries or pasta dishes to which sugars have been added	Noodles , rice, potatoes

Fruit juices, lemonades, all cola products, alcohol (wine, sparkling wine, liqueurs, beer), fruit tea	Mineral water, coffee, milk, tea without aromas, herbal tea
Fruit yoghurt, fruit butter milk etc.	Cheese without sugar, cottage cheese, natural yoghurt, eggs
Aromas	Fats (oil, butter, margarine)
Spices with prohibited sugars.	
Chocolate, cakes, pastries, ice cream, marzipan, fruit gum	snacks without added sugar: rice waffles, salt sticks
Breaded finished products	Fish, meat, poultry and eggs
Peppers, cabbage, tomatoes	Asparagus, salad cucumbers, chicory, spinach, leaf salad, avocados

Apples, pears, cherries, plums, mangoes, watermelons, kiwis, grapes, dried fruits, pineapples

8. What are sweeteners?

Sweeteners are synthetic or natural sugar substitutes, which are available in tablet form, liquid form, etc. Sweeteners have far greater sweetening power than sugars or sugar substitutes. There are, however, enormous differences in the sweetening power of sweeteners. The sweetening power of neotam is, for example, 10,000 (neotam is 10,000 times sweeter than conventional household sugar) while the sweetening power of acesulfame is 200.

The following sweeteners are authorized in the EU:

- Acesulfame
- Aspartame
- Aspartame-acesulfame salt

- Cyclamate

- Neohesperidine

- Neotam

- Saccharin

- Sucralose

- Stevia

- Thaumatin

Commercial sweeteners usually consist of saccharin and cyclamate. A combination of both sweeteners has the advantage that the slightly bitter taste of the saccharin is suppressed by the addition of cyclamate and the consumer thus tastes a pleasant sweetness.

For a long time, sweeteners were in the criticism. Again and again health risks were associated with them. However, the World Health Organization (WHO) has left the critics silent and the health safety of sweeteners fully confirmed. However, an ADI value (ADI = "Acceptable Daily Intake") was set by the WHO. This value is based on the recommended daily amount, which - assuming that sweeteners are consumed daily for a lifetime - is harmless to health. The recommended daily dose depends on the body weight and is, for example, aspartame 40 mg per kilo of body weight. This means that a woman weighing 60 kilos would have to eat more than 36 doses of an aspartame-sweetened soft drink each day to exceed the limit.

Whether one likes sweeteners or is rather critical of them is left to everyone. The following information on the advantages and disadvantages of sweeteners can in any case help to get a realistic picture of it and make a decision for itself.

Advantages of sweeteners

- Since sweeteners have a much higher sweetening power than sugars or sugar substitutes, they are automatically reduced. Thus, minimal amounts are needed to achieve the same sweetening power as sugar.

- While sugar is caries-promoting, sweeteners cannot be metabolized by the mouth flora and therefore do not provide caries for food.

- Sweeteners contain almost no energy, so by their use calories can be saved and weight gain cannot be actively encouraged.

- In addition, sweeteners do not trigger a glycemic reaction, so diabetics can take sweeteners without hesitation.

- Except for aspartame and thaumatin, sweeteners can be easily heated. This means that sweeteners are suitable as sugar substitutes for cooking and baking.

Disadvantages of sweeteners

- After animal experiments, the accusation was repeatedly expressed that sweetener is carcinogenic, i.e. carcinogenic, at very high doses. However, scientists agree today that the risk in normal doses is insignificant.

- Sweetener has been said to have an appetizing effect in the past. For example, it has been reported in the media that sweetener is used in pig fattening. Today it is known that the link between pig fattening and sweetener is attributed to legends. Pigs have different taste buds than humans. Saccharin is the only sweetener that affects humans and animals. In fact, saccharin is used for piglets until the fourth month. However, this is not done to boost their hunger, but to wean the piglet from the sweet milk to the (partial) bitter food. Fat pigs have nothing to do with sweetener.

• Last but not least: sweeteners are lacking in weight compared to sugar. For this reason, sweeteners in food technology are brought to a corresponding volume with so-called fillers (inulin, fructose and sugar alcohols). Due to the lack of weight, it is difficult to process sweeteners in the kitchen, for example, when baking.

9. What are sugar substitutes?

Whether maltitol, mannitol, isomalt, lactitol, sorbitol, xylitol or erythritol - the list of sugar substitutes is long. Sugar substitutes are sweet-tasting carbohydrates, which are obtained, for example, from fruits and vegetables, but are basically less sweet than sugars. Sugar substitutes are used by diabetics because they can be metabolized without raising the insulin level. From a health perspective, sugar substitutes are safe.

Sugar substitutes are basically available in powder form for the household. However, the use of sugar substitutes in the food industry is far more common in the production of confectionery, desserts, sauces or pastry products.

The following sugar substitutes are authorized in the EU:

- Erythritol
- Isomalt
- Mannitol
- Maltitol
- Lactitol
- Sorbitol
- Xynotlitol

Advantages of sugar substitutes

Natural sugar substitutes are not caries-promoting, as the bacteria in the plaque cannot digest the sugar substitutes. In the context of some studies conducted in Finland, it has been shown that regular consumption of xylitol (in the form of sweets or chewing gum) can even prevent the development of caries. For this reason, sugar substitutes are often used in toothpaste or chewing gum.

• A further advantage of sugar substitutes is that these have only a small influence on the blood glucose level and are metabolized without insulin. Therefore, sugar substitutes are also suitable for diabetics. Sugar substitutes have 2.4 calories per gram. This means that sugar substitutes are on average 40 percent below the caloric content of sugar.

• Last but not least: The volume of sugar substitutes corresponds to that of sugar, so that they can be processed in the kitchen similar to sugar.

Disadvantages of sugar substitutes

Sugar substitutes usually have only half as many calories as sugar, but they have about half the sweetening power, like sugar. So you have to use twice as much to get a similar result as with sugar.

In principle, sugar substitutes are harmless from a health perspective. However, since sugar substitutes cannot be absorbed completely in the small intestine, they enter the large intestine, where they absorb water and stimulate intestinal activity. Flatulence, diarrhea, and irritable bowel syndrome may result. However, here no general flat-rate judgment can be made since each human being reacts differently to sugar substitutes. Products that contain more than 10% of sugar substitutes and which may potentially lead to flatulence or diarrhea must be marked accordingly. According to the legislature, the phrase "can have a laxative effect on excessive consumption".

Agave syrup as an alternative to sugar

Agave syrup is obtained from agaves, as the name is easily recognizable. The agave is a Central American cactus, from which tequila is made. Compared to honey, agave syrup is more fluid and more soluble, but has a stronger sweetening power than honey. Agave syrup is mainly made in Mexico.

Agave juice is especially used by vegans as a sweetener to avoid honey or sugar. Depending on the sweetness, the agave syrup has a different color. So there is the almost transparent Agave syrup, which has only a very light, sweetish touch, but basically tasted almost neutral. The amber colored syrup has a stronger caramel note, which shows itself in its full strength in the dark syrup variant.

Advantages of Agave Syrup as an alternative to sugar

• The agave nectar taken from the agaves, which is finally processed into agave juice, consists largely of fructose and glucose, the proportion of fruit sugar being significantly higher than 80%. Since the glycemic index (GI) of fruit sugar is extremely low, the enjoyment of the agave syrup has little effect on the blood glucose level. The glycemic load of Agave juice is among the lowest among all sweeteners.

• Since Agave syrup is fast dissolving, it can be used well for the rounding of salad dressings or for the sweetening of cold or hot drinks. But also as a bread spread, for baking or sweetening muesli.

• A further advantage is the stronger sweetening power and the lower energy density of Agave juice. While 100g of cane sugar provides 387 calories, 100g Agave provides "only" 304 calories.

• When agaves are processed into viscous syrup, trace elements, minerals and secondary crops are preserved.

• Agave syrup is available everywhere. Whether in the supermarket, in drugstore stores, over the Internet. So you do not have to search for a long time to find something.

Disadvantages of Agave as an alternative to sugar

• The high proportion of fruit sugar in the Agave can lead to intolerance with fructose intolerance, which usually results in abdominal pain, flatulence, irritable bowel syndrome or nausea.

• Also, excessive consumption of fructose can lead to overweight and obesity, resulting in decreased glucose tolerance as well as the increased formation of urea.

• In this context, it should be emphasized that the increased intake of fructose via industrially manufactured foods promotes the storage of fats in the adipose tissue and in the liver as well as obesity since high amounts of fructose influence hormonal weight regulation. The Federal Institute for Risk Assessment therefore advises not to use fructose as a sugar substitute in industrially manufactured foods. In particular, diabetics should avoid increased consumption of foodstuffs contained in fruit.

Maple syrup as an alternative to sugar

Maple Syrup is a natural sweetener that involuntarily brings two associations: Canada and Pancakes. However, maple syrup is of course much more versatile to use than just for pancakes. Whether for baking, natural yoghurt, waffles or on ice - maple syrup gives desserts a slightly caramel, nutty note.

Maple syrup is a thickened juice extracted from Canadian maple trees and contains, besides the main ingredient, sucrose, also minerals, proteins, apple acid, glucose, fructose and water.

Maple syrup is a pure natural product. It can be used just like conventional sugars. Depending on the product, the sweetening power of maple syrup is between 60 and 70% of conventional industrial sugar. The translucence of the maple provides information about its quality. Grade A is very bright and translucent and has the best quality, while Grade D has a very strong, strong flavor and is of lower quality.

Advantages of maple syrup as an alternative to sugar

- Maple syrup is a natural product and should be dissolved in a tea or a hot milk, help with sleeping disorders and have an anti-inflammatory effect.

● Maple syrup has fewer calories than sugar: While 100g of sugar has 387 calories, it brings maple syrup with the same amount to 276 calories.

● Not to forget, of course, that maple syrup is available everywhere.

Disadvantages of maple syrup as an alternative to sugar

● For people with diabetes, maple syrup is not suitable.

● When sweetening with maple syrup, it should be considered that this can be an expensive fun.

● In Europe the term "maple syrup" is not protected, so the thickened juice is sometimes mixed with sugar water and diluted with it. when a sugar-free diet this can be very annoying - so make sure to take a look at the ingredients list.

• It is also important to remember that the sweetness of maple syrup is lower and that more maple syrup must be used in order to achieve the same sweetness as industrial sugar

Apple juice as an alternative to sugar

Apple juice is basically nothing but highly concentrated apple juice, which has been heated and boiled to a viscous mass. Thus, apple juice has an intense apple aroma and is therefore suitable for the refining of desserts, muesli, compote and salad dressings.

Apple juice is quite easy to make. Simply squeeze the juice from six kilos of apples and boil it for about three hours at medium heat to about one fifth of the original quantity. Then drain through a sieve, fill into sterilized bottles and close airtight. The apple juice obtained from it is stable for about one year.

Advantages of apple juice as an alternative to sugar

- Apple juice is a natural sweetener that has a slightly lower sweetness than sugar and has an average of about 35% less calories.

- In mineral juice, minerals, trace elements and secondary crops are preserved.

- When looking at sugar substitutes from a sustainable perspective, apple juice is convincing in comparison to other sweeteners, as apple juices can be produced without problems and / or from regional production.

Disadvantages of apple juice as an alternative to sugar

• Apple juice contains a high concentration of fruit sugar. Those suffering from fructose intolerance or malabsorption should therefore dispense with apple juice, since this can lead to flatulence or diarrhea.

• A disadvantage is that apple juice is about 83% sugar. As a result of boiling, high amounts of glucose, sucrose and fruit sugar remain in the apple juice, but the proportion of minerals and vitamins is very low.

• Due to its sticky, tough consistency, apple juice is quickly caught in the tooth spaces and can thus be tooth-damaging.

• If you want to use apple juice for baking, remember that apple juice has a higher moisture content than sugar and therefore the amount of liquid used in the recipe should be reduced accordingly in order to achieve a good baking result.

Aspartame as an alternative to sugar

Aspartame belongs to the synthetic sweeteners group, which are produced in the laboratory, and is often used by the food industry in chewing gum, confectionery, ready-to-serve meals, soft drinks and dairy products.

Aspartame was repeatedly criticized, as it was suspected of causing cancer. This was enough reason for the European Food Safety Authority (EFSA) to get to the bottom of the matter and to examine aspartame once again for health-damaging risks.

The trigger was an Italian study conducted in 2010, which concluded that mice developed tumors after consumption of aspartame. Furthermore, it was stated that the risk of miscarriage with daily consumption of aspartame is increased. Critics of these studies admitted, however, that the standards under which the studies were conducted had nothing to do with the normal consumption of aspartame and there was a maximum dosage of aspartame.

The EU limit value for aspartame was fixed at 40 mg / kg body weight. This means in practice that a person weighing 60 kilos would have to drink more than 36 doses of an aspartame-sweetened lemonade per day to exceed the limit.

Advantages of aspartame as an alternative to sugar

- Aspartame has an energy content of 17 KJ/g, which is very low compared to sugar. If you replace sugar with aspartame, you can save significantly calories.

- The sweetening power of aspartame is two times as high as that of sugar, so much lower amounts are needed to produce the same sweetness as sugar.

- Aspartame is suitable for diabetes.

• In addition, aspartame does not promote caries.

Disadvantages of aspartame as an alternative to sugar

• People suffering from phenylketonuria under metabolic disease are not allowed to consume aspartame because they cannot degrade the amino acid phenylalanine - a component of aspartame.

• For people who want to eat as naturally as possible, a synthetically produced sweetener is, of course, anything but recommended.

Bananas as an alternative to sugar

Banana trees are among the oldest cultivated plants in the world. Besides maize, sugar and flour, the banana is one of the most important world trade products.

Compared to other fruits, bananas do not just shine with a high vitamin content. However, bananas also contain important minerals such as potassium, magnesium, phosphorus, iron, manganese and copper in addition to water (70%), fiber and sugar.

Benefits of bananas as an alternative to sugar

- Since the proportion of fructose contained in bananas is less than the proportion of glucose, the body does not recognize fructose. Bananas are therefore not a problem even for people with fructose intolerance.

Disadvantages of bananas as an alternative to sugar

- As the ARD documentation "Cheap, Cheap, Banana" showed, the price for bananas has not increased for 20 years. Inadequate work and social standards in the producing countries are the result. Unfortunately, too few consumers are resorting to organic bananas or fair trade traded bananas.

- Bananas lead to a very mild sweetness. For example, if you like it a bit sweeter when baking, bananas will not come too far.

Dates as an alternative to sugar

Dates either pure as a dry bob or in a bacon coat, dates are very popular here. The fact that they can also easily be taken as sugar substitutes or in the form of dates syrup, is probably unknown to many.

Dates are the fruits of the date palm, mainly in Egypt, Saudi Arabia and Iran. Until the first dates can be reaped, one must be very patient: the date palm carries the coveted fruits only from the tenth year.

Dates are not without reason called the bread of the desert. Because dates provide the body with energy quickly. They consist of 70% of carbohydrates, fructose and glucose in equal parts. Also, dates contain important minerals such as potassium, magnesium, iron, phosphorus and calcium.

As an alternative sweetener to cane sugar dates are either minced or in the form of dates syrup. For this purpose, the dates are pitted and placed in water. Subsequently, the pulp is boiled to a thick liquid mass.

Advantages of dates as an alternative to sugar

• Dates are digestive. In addition, the high content of pantothenic acid (vitamin B5) stimulates energy metabolism in the body cells.

• As dates quickly provide energy and quickly satisfy the hunger between them, they are suitable not only for sweetening, but also as a snack between or for fast energy supply for athletes.

• Dates are best combined with a few nuts and fresh fruit for sweetening the morning cereal. But date also makes a difference in Christmas baking or fruit salad.

• Dates are generally suitable for diabetics. However, diabetics should eat only three to four dates a day.

• The energy density of dates is 282 calories per 100g, well below the calorie content of sugar, which is 387 calories per 100g sugar.

Disadvantages of dates as an alternative to sugar

• Anyone suffering from fructose intolerance or malabsorption should refrain from using dates, since these have a high propor-

tion of fruit sugar and thus lead to flatulence or diarrhea.

Coconut nectar as an alternative to sugar

Coconut nectar or coconut blossom nectar
is produced from the juice of the coconut blos-
soms. Coconut nectar replaces sugar 1: 1 and is
just like sugar or sweetener for cooking and
baking. Coconut nectar is reminiscent of caramel. The nectar is therefore versatile - whether
in the coffee, fruit salad or for the refining of
salads, sauces or Asian dishes.

Benefits of coconut nectar as an alternative to sugar

• The glycemic load of coconut nectar is
very low, meaning that after the consumption of coconut nectar the blood glucose
level rise up more slowly. Thus, the glycemic index of coconut nectar is 35 while that

of refined sugar is 80. This has the advantage, among other things, that the blood glucose level after consumption of coconut blossom nectar does not ride roller coaster and therefore one feels longer saturated.

- Compared to brown cane sugar, coconut nectar has twice as much iron, four times as much magnesium and ten times as much zinc.

- Those who suffer from fructose intolerance and therefore have to be cautious with honey or agave donuts, might have found a suitable sweetener with coconut nectar, which contains relatively little fructose with 10% fructose.

Disadvantages of coconut nectar as an alternative to sugar

- 250ml coconut nectar is expensive.

- Since coconut nectar is handmade by Asian small farmers and has to go a long way to western countries from Southeast Asia, one should consider from a sustainable point of view two times, whether it is actually coconut nectar.

Honey as an alternative to sugar

Honey is the oldest sweetener and is certainly one of the most common alternatives to avoid industrial sugar. Honey comes from flower nectar or honeydew and is produced by honeybees and some ant species for their own food supply. It should be stored cool, dark and in a dry environment. This ensures that the aromas and enzymes remain intact.

Honey consists mainly of fructose (depending on honey type between 28 and 45%), glucose (21 to 40%) and water (about 18%). Minerals, enzymes, phytonutrients and vitamins play a subordinate role. What is amazing is that nowhere in the world is so much honey eaten as in Germany. Per person, we eat Germans on average just under 1.5 kilos per year.

Advantages of honey as an alternative to sugar

- Due to the high proportion of fructose, the sweetness of honey is higher than that of cane sugar.

- A further advantage is the lower energy density of honey. While bringing 100g of cane sugar to 387 calories, 100g of honey "only" beats with 300 calories.

- Honey is often called an anti-inflammatory effect. The fact is that honey is therefore used for medical purposes, for example in wounds treated with honey pads. The fact that this is a sterile product, which has nothing to do with the honey from the supermarket, many forget.

• A great advantage of honey is, of course, that it is available everywhere, in contrast to many other sugary substitutes (erythritol).

Disadvantages of honey as an alternative to sugar

• Honey, which consists of exactly the same constituents as sugar, namely, fructose and glucose, can penetrate well into the interdental spaces. With its sticky consistency it can spread well and long on the tooth surface and has the same effect with regard to caries exactly the same or in a more harmful effect than sugar.

• The Robert Koch Institute recommends that babies under 12 months should not be given honey, since honey can encourage the spores of certain bacteria which can lead to symptoms of paralysis by the pathogen Clostridium Botulinum. In the case of children and adults, on the other hand, honey is absolutely safe.

• While conventional industrial sugar is commonly considered artificial, honey is often considered a natural product. It is, however, forgotten that the main components of honey and sugar are very similar. Therefore, honey should be measured.

• Due to the high fructose content, honey can lead to diarrhea in fructosemal absorption, that is to say fructose intolerance.

• If honey is heated above 40 ° C, important ingredients are lost. Therefore, you should refrain from cooking with honey.

Rice Syrup as an alternative to sugar

Rice syrup is obtained by dissolving ground rice in water and boiling it into syrup. The rice starch is split into multiple sugars, malt sugar and glucose.

While rice syrup has been used as a sweetener in Asian cuisine for a long time, it is now enjoying increasing popularity in our clime. Rice syrup has a nutty-caramel flavor and is therefore perfect for home-made nut nougat creams, but of course also for the refining of desserts, milk dishes and muesli. The consistency and color of rice syrup resembles that of honey, so that rice syrup is also often referred to as rice honey.

Advantages of Rice Syrup as an alternative to sugar

- Rice syrup contains numerous natural minerals such as iron, calcium and magnesium, which are important for bones, muscles and blood formation.

- Furthermore, Rice syrup does not contain fructose, so that the syrup offers the ideal sugar supplement for fructose intolerance or fructose malabsorption.

• Rice syrup also offers a good alternative to honey for vegans.

• With a share of just under 21% of long-chained multiple sugars, sugar intake in the blood is delayed, so that the blood glucose level rises slowly and the feeling of saturation lasts longer.

Disadvantages of rice syrup as an alternative to sugar

• Rice syrup comes with 316 calories on a similar calorie balance as cane sugar, which is at 387 calories.

• However, since the sweetening power of rice syrup is lower than that of sugar, more rice syrup must be used to achieve the same sweetness. The (few) saved calories can quickly land on the hips.

• If you want to use rice syrup for baking, consider that rice syrup has a higher moisture content than sugar and therefore the amount of liquid used in the recipe should be reduced by about 10% in order to achieve a good baking result.

Sorbitol as an alternative to sugar

Sorbitol is a sugar substitute, which was originally obtained from rowan berries, the fruits of the mountain ash. As an intermediate of the carbohydrate metabolism, sorbitol is also present in many core nuts (e.g. plums, apricots, peaches). Dried fruits, such as dried peaches or apricots, contain about five times as much sorbitol as fresh peaches or apricots.

Sorbitol is industrially produced by corn and wheat starch. Today, sorbitol is often used in diabetic foods, sugar-free ice cream, confectionery, lozenges, chewing gum and toothpaste. Often, however, sorbitol is also used in the food industry to protect food from drying out.

Advantages of sorbitol as an alternative to sugar

• Sorbitol contains 2.4 kcal / g and thus has a lower energy content than conventional household sugar.

• Sorbitol is also suitable for diabetics because no insulin is needed for metabolism in the body.

Disadvantages of sorbitol as an alternative to sugar

• The sweetening power of sorbitol is about 40 to 60% of the sweetening power of conventional household sugar. Thus, more sorbitol is needed to achieve the same sweetness.

• Sorbitol can cause diarrhea, stomach pain and flatulence if excessive consumption (more than 50g / day). For this reason, any food containing more than 10% sorbitol must be labeled with the phrase "may have a laxative effect when consumed excessively".

- If sorbitol is incompatible, sorbitol cannot be digested in the small intestine. In this case, one should completely dispense with food containing sorbitol. Whether a sorbitol intolerance is present can be diagnosed by a breath test.

- If fructose intolerance is present, the consumption of sorbitol-containing foods should also be reduce as sorbitol reduces the absorption capacity of fructose in the stomach even further.

Stevia as an alternative to sugar

A sweet and honeyed herb native to South America now also conquers the market. Stevia rebaudiana, short Stevia! If you want to drastically reduce your sugar consumption, but do not necessarily want to use the sweeteners produced in the laboratory, you will have a real pleasure at Stevia.

The leaves of the stevia plant have been used for more than 500 years by the aborigines of Brazil and Paraguay as a remedy as well as for the sweetening of teas and foodstuffs. The main producer of the sweet corn is now China.

Stevia is available in tablets, capsules, powders or in liquid form. Stevia is not only available, but is used more and more by the food industry and is already found today in fruit spreads, sweets, drinks and even ketchup.

Advantages of Stevia as an alternative to sugar

- Actually it sounds too good to be true: Stevia has no influence on the blood glucose level and is therefore suitable for diabetics.

- Stevia has, depending on the product, the 300 times the sweetness of sugar.

- In addition, Stevia is not carcinogenic, so it is not caries-promoting.

- Another great advantage: Stevia is almost free of calories.

- In addition, Stevia is available everywhere in the supermarket, in drugstore shops, but also in the internet, in powdered, liquid or tablet form, in contrast to many other sugar generators (erythritol, xylitol).

Disadvantages of stevia as an alternative to sugar

- The commercially available stevia is not a natural product because it consists of isolated steviolglycosides, the sweet-tasting chemical compounds of the stevia plant. These are extracted in complex chemical processes. A natural product definitely looks different.

• Test persons partly report a long-lasting, bitter aftertaste when consuming stevia products. This is caused by the activation of the bitter taste receptors on the tongue. Because of this peculiar taste, which is partly described as bitter, partly as liquorice-like, most products are not sweetened exclusively with stevia, but to a certain extent also with sugar or other sweeteners.

• When buying stevia sweetened foods or beverages, you should take a look at the nutrition table. Stevia's proprietary taste is often used by industry to avoid the flavor of liquorice and to remain below the prescribed level for stevia, as the European Food Safety Authority recommends not consuming a maximum of four milligrams of stevia equivalent per kilogram of body weight.

• Basically you can bake well with stevia, since it is heat stable. However, dosing is a problem because dough varieties where sugar is a major ingredient (cake or biscuit) differ enormously in volume and consistency when sweetened with stevia instead of sugar. For example, a loose-air stirring dough with Stevia is quickly dry and flat.

Xylitol as an alternative to sugar

Xylitol is a sugar substitute that is found as a natural sugar alcohol in the bark of some species of wood (e.g. birch) as well as in a variety of fruit and vegetable varieties.

Advantages of xylitol as an alternative to sugar

• So abstruse it may sound for a sugar exchange: Xylitol has a cariostatic and anti-cariogenic effect. This means that the caries bacteria (Streptococcus mutans) in the mouth cannot metabolize xylitol and thus die. But not only that! Xylitol can even significantly reduce the number of caries bacteria in the saliva as well as in the tooth plaque, i.e., caries-reducing. For example, two studies have shown that xylitol is highly effective in reducing caries. Anyone who takes about 5 to 10g of xylitol in the form of pastilles or gum per day is optimally positioned. Also mouthwashes with xylitol are very effective.

* Xylitol has a similar sweetness as conventional sugars but has a 40% lower nutritional value than sucrose.

* Since xylitol is metabolized insulin-independent, i.e. the insulin level is only slightly influenced, xylitol is suitable for diabetics. For this reason, xylitol also plays an important role in a carbohydrate-reduced diet.

* Xylitol is the only sugar substitute which is very well tolerated even in metabolic defects.

• In contrast to some other sugar substitutes, xylitol is permitted for some foods without a limit on the quantity.

Disadvantages of xylitol as an alternative to sugar

• Xylitol can also be produced from glucose, for example from corn starch. Genetically modified maize is often used for this purpose. Since the glucose is an intermediate product, there is no need for labeling in this case. Of course, cultivation of genetically engineered maize is still relatively low in Europe, especially compared to the USA. However, when purchasing xylitol, it is not possible to rule out the use of genetically modified maize.

• Xylitol has a slightly lower sweetness than sugar. Thus, a little more must be taken to achieve the same degree of sweetness.

• Xylitol can have a laxative effect and an exfoliating effect.

• To date, the reference sources of xylitol are mostly restricted to the Internet.

Sugar beet syrup as an alternative to sugar

The sugar beet syrup, which is also known as beet or beet juice, is obtained from the juice of the sugar beet, as the name is easily recognizable. To this end, the sugar beet juice is heated without the use of additives, pressed and finally thickened to form a syrup. This produces a dark brown, viscous mass, which is often used as a spread of bread, but also for cooking or baking due to its malty caramel character, and is suitable, for example, for refining sauces or for sweetening wafers or pancakes.

Advantages of sugar beet syrup as an alternative to sugar

- Besides sugar, sugar beet syrup contains, among other things, protein, iron, magnesium, zinc, potassium and folic acid. Thus the daily requirement for iron can be covered with 100 g sugar beet syrup.

- Additives such as flavorings, flavor enhancers or stabilizers can be a long time in sugar beet syrup since sugar beet syrup is the natural response to synthetically produced sweeteners.

- Sugar beet syrup is one of the basic foods, so that it can be used as part of a basement for the deacidification of the body.

Disadvantages of sugar beet syrup as an alternative to sugar

- With 299 calories per 100g, sugar beet syrup cannot be described as a low-calorie alternative to sugar (by comparison, sugar has 387 calories / 100g).

Also, the sweetness of sugar beet syrup is lower, so that more sugar beet syrup is needed to achieve the same sweetness as that of sugar.

10. Life without sugar - but how?

That the sugar portion in chocolate is considerable and milk chocolate is not infrequently more than 50% sugar, is not really surprising. However, many people are not aware of the fact that salad dressings, pastries, sausages or dairy products also contain sugars. And so the amounts of sugar we ingest every day are far greater than we think.

Excessive consumption of sugar can lead to stomach problems, loss of concentration and lack of energy. Of course, diabetes, obesity, and the associated increased risk of developing cancer, cardiovascular disease and dementia are also associated with an uncontrolled consumption of sugar. Those who are actively trying to minimize their consumption of sugar actively are doing something for their health. But how do I reduce my sugar consumption? Here are 5 easy ways to reduce your sugar consumption.

1. Do not eat sweets!

Actually, it is obvious: If you want to reduce your sugar consumption, you should do without confectionery sweets, biscuits, wine gum, chocolate, and muesli or ice cream. I advise you not to buy any sweets. For only few of us possess the necessary willpower and manage to put the once-opened bar of chocolate back into the cupboard. At the beginning of the diet, it may be advisable to take a critical look at the sweet supplies at home and give them to friends and acquaintances.

If you get appetite for sweets, you should try to distract yourself first. A walk around the block or a phone call with your best friend can sometimes be distraction enough. If all this does not help, drink a large glass of water first. Thirst is often confused with hunger. Also a mouthwash with xylitol can be helpful. This has two advantages: the palate comes to benefit of sweetness and you profit from the cariostatic and anticariogenic effect of xylitol. If the sweet temptations still persist, try a piece of fruit, which you deliberately enjoy. Only in the last step should you grab the chocolate.

Tip: Also sweet bread spreads and jam should preferably not be bought any more. In a glass of Nutella, you'll find a total of 78 pieces of cube sugar, in a glass jam of 102 pieces.

2. Do not drink sugary drinks!

Those who decide to minimize their consumption of sugar are most likely thinking of chocolate, pastries and sweets. The sugar content of beverages surprised many. That a large bottle of cola contains 53 pieces of cube sugar is known to many. But what about iced tea, fruit juices or wellness drinks? One liter of ice tea contains up to 24 pieces of cube sugar, the healthy sounding wellness water up to 17 pieces of sugar. Caution is also advised with orange juice or apple juice. For example, one liter of apple juice contains about 100g of sugar, which corresponds to 17 pieces of cube sugar.

Our energy supply should not exceed 10% sugar per day. After half a liter of apple juice, this value would have been reached. I therefore recommend not to buy any sugary drinks at all. The fluid supply should be covered by water and herbal teas.

Tip: Of course you should deal with alcoholic beverages with caution.

3. Take a look at the nutritional values!

Firstly, it is important to be aware of where sugar is contained. Before you put food into the shopping cart, you should get used to taking a look at the nutritional values. Here, the nutritional table on the back of the package provides a comprehensive overview. For you, the term "carbohydrates - sugars" is interesting in this context.

Also interesting is a look at the ingredients list. Here the normal household sugar, the so-called sucrose, can hide behind many names. Whether fructose, glucose, dextrose, maltose, molasses, lactose, invert sugar syrup or matrodextrin, all of these terms stand for sugars. The actual quantity of sugar is thus concealed and is only recognizable to the consumer at second sight. Good to know, because only the few are aware of hidden sugar falls.

By the way, the World Health Organization recommends taking a maximum of 25 grams of sugar per day. This corresponds to about 6 teaspoons of sugar. Critically, the WHO sees all above as free sugar, i.e. conventional industrial sugar, which is added to food and beverages, but also honey, syrup or the sugar contained in fruit juices.

4. Grip yourself to the cooking spoon!

Pastries, muffins and biscuits contain lots of sugar, no question. A raisin worm from the baker contains a total of 19 pieces of cube sugar. Sweet pastry should therefore be avoided as far as possible. For example, you can simply reduce the amount of sugar indicated in the recipe, or you can completely dispense with sugar and choose an alternative.

It is a positive thing to consciously deal with sugars, that our taste buds are sensitized again, and that we are again more aware of the taste of the food. For excessive consumption of sugar leaves our taste buds dull. In order to feel the same degree of sweetening, we must eat more and more sugar over time.

Tip: If you are accustomed to a meal with a sweet dessert, you should try it alternatively with an espresso and a piece of cheese and a little fig. Or simply move the dessert simply by half an hour backwards.

5. Learn to find hidden sugar sources! Caution with extract flour!

White flour products are usually rapidly metabolized, resulting in a rapid increase in insulin levels. The starch contained in the extracted flour is converted by the body into energy in the form of sugar. If the proportion of white flour products is reduced, the proportion of sugar is automatically reduced.

Now and again to dispense with white flour products is not only helpful to limit the consumption of sugar, but also helps to lose a few superfluous pounds.

Attention for dairy products!

Caution is also needed with dairy products. A small fruit yoghurt from the supermarket contains 8 diced sugar. The small yogurt drinks marketed as a probiotic, which supposedly strengthen the defense or have a positive effect on digestion, contain 4 to 5 pieces of cube sugar.

Therefore: If you have appetite for yogurt, take a look at the nutritional values. Usually, it should be a natural yogurt, soy yogurt, kefir or Greek yogurt. With a few fresh berries or other fresh fruits of the season you will surely miss nothing.

11. 9 tips for a life without sugar

You want to reduce your sugar consumption to a minimum or from now on completely without sugar? With the following tips you can create the ideal conditions for a (almost) sugar-free life. Here you go:

1. Start the day!

Make sure you allow your body at least 8 hours of rest at night. Lack of sleep or the resulting lack of energy leads to an increased craving for sugar. As US researchers from the University of California found out in Los Angeles, sleep deprivation encourages hunger. Those who suffers from chronic insomnia has an increased risk of being overweight. So do not make the night a day, but allow yourself and your body enough sleep and rest!

2. Start the day with a healthy breakfast!

If you start the day with a healthy breakfast, you will have to struggle less with sudden hunger pangs or cravings. A homemade muesli made from oatmeal, crunchy nuts and fresh fruit can do wonders. If you should decide to buy a ready-to-eat cereal from the supermarket, please take a look at the list of ingredients to see if the muesli contains sugar, glucose or other sugars. Breakfast cereals consist partly of 40% sugar. So look!

By the way, the school of thought that breakfast is the most important meal of the day has now been disproved by nutritionists. So if you do not want to eat in the morning, you can eat a banana. So the blood glucose level is raised, which boosts our performance and lets us start the day with energy.

3. Have regular exercise!

People who move regularly feel fitter, healthier and more energetic. In addition, candy is reduced by sport and sufficient sunlight.

One thing is clear: those who practice sports burn their calories during training. In addition, the body empties messengers - so to speak, body-borne appetite suppressants - which signal saturation to the body, while the appetizing hormone ghrelin does not increase as a result of sporting activity. So you have a double reason to engage sport, do not you?

4. Take 5 small meals a day to you!

If you limit yourself daily to 3 meals, there is the risk that the blood sugar level drops so much that you get hot hunger and then quickly grab a sweet snack. It is therefore better to eat

5 small meals daily consisting of complex carbohydrates, healthy fats and proteins. Thus, the blood glucose level remains stable all day, and hot shower attacks can not occur at all.

5. Prevent untreated, full-fledged foods!

If foodstuffs have been processed in a highly industrial way, almost 100% safety sugar or sugar substitutes are found in the list of ingredients. Whether in ketchup, sausage, vinegar cucumbers, red cabbage or potato or herring salad - the supermarket shelves are full of hidden sugar sources.

You are doing a lot of good to your body, if you prefer untreated, full-fledged foods, and ready-made meals are an absolute exception. This also applies to salad dressings, which generally contain 10 to 15% sugar. So why not grab the ladle yourself? In any case, you should take a look at the nutritional values in the supermarket and convince yourself that the product of your choice does not contain sugar.

Special caution should be exercised:

- Fruit and vegetable preserves

- Fast food and ready-to-serve foods (here sugar is often used as a flavor carrier)

- Soft drinks

- Breakfast cereals and muesli

- Fruit juices

- fruit yoghurt

- Bakery products

- Ketchup, sauces and dressings from the supermarket

- Sweet spreads

- granola bar

- Low-fat and light products (sugar is often used as a flavor carrier)

6. Define what is sugar-free for you!

The more accurate you define at the beginning of your diet change, what you want to do in the next weeks, months and perhaps even years, the easier will be the loss of sugar. Do you want to do without refined sugar or honey, Stevia and Agave syrup? What about fructose and lactose? Think about what is realistic and practical for you in everyday life. If the goals are too high, there is a risk that the drastic sugar removal will not be long lasting in everyday life. Therefore, first of all, set small, but realistic goals, which one gradually increases!

7. Remove the sweets from your household!

There are people who can enjoy a bit of chocolate and then leave the opened chocolate pack for the coming weeks in the closet. However, if you have to empty the entire package as soon as it is opened, you should avoid such sugar traps from the start by banishing sweets and sugar from the household at the start of the sugar-free diet. You should not make it harder than it is anyway.

You will notice: If you nourish yourself and naturally wean the body of sugar, you will gradually lose less and more sweetness, because this is the only way to give your taste buds the chance to regain even smaller amounts of sugar.

Whoever, find it difficult to dispense with sugar completely from today to tomorrow, should reduce the amount of sugar slowly. How about halving the sugar in morning coffee? Or, when baking, just take half of the indicated sugar and - if necessary - sweeten the rest with honey, banana, birch sugar or dates?

8. Replace old habits with new ones!

Often it is the habit that makes us not to follow through the ambitious plans. Whether it is after the lunch, for the afternoon coffee or whether the television is only half as much fun without those hot beloved jelly bears. If you decides for a more conscious handling of sugar, you should take a critical look at your habits and look for alternatives. Perhaps there are healthier and, above all, sugar-free snacks, with which snacking does not have to be quite a thing of the past, but with which one is doing something good for himself and his body!

9. Write a Nutrition Book!

A nutritional diary cannot only help to critically examine the eating habits and to expose possible sugar traps. If you include your mood and your starting weight as well as the possible successes of the sugar zap (better body feeling, better skin condition, etc.), the dietary diary in a weak minute may also help to overcome possible hot weather attacks.

12. Recipes with Little or No sugar for breakfast

Anyone who likes to start the day in the morning is confronted with a problem when he decides to cut down on his sugar consumption drastically or even to forego sugar.

Not surprisingly, popular breakfast favors such as Nutella (a glass of 78 cube sugar) or jam (a glass of 72 cube sugar) are true sugar bombs. But what are the alternatives? The fact that you want to embark on sugar-free diet does not automatically mean that you have to start from now with liver sausage and scrambled eggs, I show you here with a few delicious suggestions and prescriptions without sugar.

It goes without sugar!

True sweet addicts will hardly be lured by a hearty liver sausage in the morning. Therefore, the good news: If you want to eat without sugar, you do not have to miss a sweet breakfast in the morning. However, there are some things to consider:

If it is absolutely a jam bread or bread, you can spread the bread with some fresh cheese, so that the jam layer is a bit thinner and the sugar content is somewhat reduced. Disadvantage of the jam is, however, that the blood-sugar level rises to the height and plummet again soon afterwards. Thus, a growling stomach and lack of concentration capacity are preprogrammed. A healthy, full-fledged muesli is the ideal start to the day. The coffee or tea should preferably be enjoyed without sugar.

Sugar-free breakfasts:

Recipes for spreads and jam without sugar:

- Recipe for strawberry jam without sugar
- Recipe for cherry jam without sugar
- Recipe for a nut-nougat cream without sugar
- Recipe for plum without sugar

Recipes for Pancakes and Co. Without Sugar:

- Recipe for banana oatmeal pancakes without sugar
- Recipe for banana pancakes without sugar
- Recipe for blueberry pancakes without sugar
- Recipe for gluten-free blueberry pancakes without sugar
- Recipe for a pannukaku without sugar

Recipes for muffins and scones without sugar:

- Recipe for apple and carrot muffins without sugar

- Recipe for apple full grain muffins without sugar

- Recipe for banana muffins without sugar

- Recipe for blueberry without sugar

- Recipe for oat-blue muffins without sugar

- Recipe for an oat flake raspberry chick without sugar

- Recipe for chocolate scones without sugar

Recipes for muesli and co. Without sugar:

- Recipe for a sugar-free apple oatmeal slurry

- Recipe for crispy apple muesli without sugar

- Recipe for a Chia-raspberry yoghurt without sugar

- Recipe for Chia-Overnight Oats with Mangomus

- Recipe for a fitness muesli without sugar

- Recipe for a crunchy sugar without sugar

- Recipe for an almond blueberry chia pudding without sugar

- Recipe for a Matcha Chia Pudding without Sugar (not suitable for children)

- Recipe for muesli without sugar

- Recipe for a sugar-free oatmeal mango muesli

- Recipe for a quinoa breakfast slurry without sugar

- Recipe for an overnight chocolate chia pudding
- Recipe for a Cinnamon Chia Pudding
- Recipe for a cinnamon crunchy without sugar

Recipes for breakfast salads and smoothie Bowls without sugar:

- Recipe for an apple-avocado fruit salad
- Recipe for an avocado citrus salad with buttermilk dressing
- Recipe for a Banana-Chocolate Smoothie Bowl
- Recipe for a Blaubeer breakfast salad
- Recipe for a Blueberry Qunioa Bowl without Sugar
- Recipe for a Chai Smoothie Bowl without sugar
- Recipe for an oatmeal quinoa salad

- Recipe for a vegan breakfast salad

- Recipe for quinoa fruit salad with honey and lime dressing

12.1. Recipe for strawberry jam without sugar

What would summer be like without strawberries? The little, red fruits have it all in itself. They are true vitamin bombs. 100g strawberries cover the daily requirement of vitamin C. And since they are 90% water, 100g strawberries have just 30 calories. Why not simply boil the strawberries to keep the summer a bit longer? Here we have a great recipe for strawberry jam. Naturally sugar free!

ingredients

- 1000g strawberries
- 2 tsp agar
- Stevia
-

preparation

1. Place the strawberries in a cooking pot and simmer until they are easily crumbled

2. Add the agar and a little stevia and simmer again for 10 to 15 minutes

3. Mix the straw mixture with a puree

4. Rinse the hot water jars hotly and place them in the still hot oven for approximately 10 minutes (with the opening upwards)

5. Now fill the strawberry jam into the sterile storage jars, close and place the jars upside down so that a vacuum is obtained

6. The strawberry jam is kept in the refrigerator for about 3 weeks.

Nutritional values

- Results: 4 glasses
- Calories: 295.5 kcal
- Fat: 4.0g
- Carbohydrates: 55.0g
- Protein: 8.0g

12.2. Recipe for cherry jam without sugar

Whoever has a cherry tree in the garden can be lucky. With this delicious cherry jam you can quickly and easily - and without sugar - preserve a piece of the unshakable summer time and enjoy on cold autumn and winter days

ingredients

- 1500g Sweet cherries
- 1 pack of Gelfix Super 3: 1
- 2 tablespoons of water
- 3 teaspoon stevia granules
- 2 tsp cinnamon
- 1 teaspoon lemon juice
- 4cl Amaretto

preparation

1. Pour the cherries together with the water, stevia, cinnamon, lemon juice and amaretto into a cooking pot

2. Let the mixture simmer for about 10 minutes, stirring constantly

3. Then add the gel mix. Let it boil again

4. Now go through the cherry mass with a blender

5. Let the jam simmer for a further 20 minutes until it becomes firm

6. Now place in hot rinsed glasses, close quickly and place on the lid. Let it cool down - done!

7. The sugar-free cherry jam is about 1 year durable.

Nutritional values

- Calories: 932.4 kcal
- Fat: 4.5g
- Carbohydrates: 203.7g
- Protein: 13.5g

12.3. Recipe for a nut-nougat cream without sugar

The hazelnut bread spreads available in the supermarket taste delicious, no question. If, however, you remember that in a glass of the said bread dumpling are up to 78 pieces of diced sugar, one can quickly get the bread stuck in the throat. This is all the better if you know how to help yourself and you can even make a sugar-free version of the nut nougat cream. With our recipe, which is really easy to put into practice, you and your children will have your true joy.

ingredients

- 150ml almond milk
- 100g hazelnuts, ground
- 4 tablespoons cocoa powder, deoiled
- Honey to taste

preparation

1. Add all the ingredients except the honey to a mixing bowl and mix to a creamy mass

2. Then sweeten with some honey

Nutritional values

- Calories: 913.2 kcal
- Fat: 62.4g
- Carbohydrates: 70.9g
- Protein: 10.3g

12.4. Recipe for plum without sugar

Plums contain besides Vitamin A and Vitamin C and E nearly all B vitamins, which is important for a healthy metabolism as well as an intact nervous system. With such a vitamin bomb, of course, all the good things done with his plums are not immediately destroyed by excessive consumption of sugar. So why not just try a recipe for plum or plums without sugar?

Preparation time:
Baking time: 120 minutes
Total time: 2 hours

ingredients

- 3000g Plums, ripe
- 1 teaspoon cinnamon
- 1 tsp cloves

preparation

1. First of all it is about the plums. These must be pitted and halved in the first step

2. Now add the plums together with the cinnamon into a sufficiently large, oven-appropriate pan or roasting pan

3. Fill the carnations into a tea-egg, which also comes into the pot.

4. Now it is said to have patience: the pot disappears (without lid) for about 2 hours at 180 ° C in the oven. Stirring occasionally

5. After 2 hours, the tea egg is removed and the mass is finely pureed with a blender

6. Rinse the hot water jars hotly and place them in the still hot

oven for approximately 10 minutes (with the opening facing upwards)

7.　　Now fill the plum mass into the sterile storage jars and set it upside down to create a vacuum

8.　　The plum is finished without sugar.

Nutritional values

- Calories: 1384.2 kcal
- Fat: 6g
- Carbohydrates: 306g
- Protein: 18g

12.5. Recipe for banana oatmeal pancakes without sugar

This variant with oatmeal and bananas may not correspond to the classic of the pancake. Delicious are the banana oatmeal pancakes but all the time! The pancakes are pure pleasure, but can also be eaten with maple syrup, some honey, cream, some hot cherries or some yogurt.

ingredients

- 60g flour
- 35g oatmeal
- 1 Banana, ripe, crushed
- 1 egg
- 3 tbsp of milk
- 2.5 EL water
- 1.5 EL agave syrup
- 1 tablespoon linseed

- 1 teaspoon Baking powder
- 1 teaspoon vanilla flavor
- 1 teaspoon sesame oil
- 1 pinch of salt

PREPARATION

1. Mix the linseed with the water and leave to soak for about 10 minutes

2. Meanwhile, crush the banana and give it together with the baking soda, the salt and the agave syrup in a mixing bowl

3. Sesame oil, egg, vanilla flavor and milk and mix the ingredients into a smooth dough

4. Now add the oatmeal, the linseed and the flour. Stir again

5. If the dough appears too viscous, add another shot of milk

6.   Heat some sesame oil in a frying pan and add the dough portionwise into the pan

7.   Bake for about 2-4 minutes and, as soon as the edges of the pancake bend, turn around and bake from the other side

12.6. Recipe for banana pancakes without sugar

Banana pancakes and banana pancakes lead to absolute enthusiasm among children (and adults). Here we have a lightning recipe for you - without sugar, of course! The mature bananas give the pancake a healthy sweetness, so that conventional industrial sugar can remain safely in the cupboard.

Preparation time: 5 minutes
Baking time:
Total time: 5 minutes

INGREDIENTS
- 150ml of milk
- 100g spelled flour
- 2 bananas, ripe
- 1 tablespoon maple syrup

- 2 tsp of baking soda
- 1 pinch of salt
- Some oil

PREPARATION

1. Add the flour, baking powder, milk, maple syrup and salt to a pancake dough

2. Cut the bananas into thin slices, set aside

3. Now heat some oil in a coated pan and add some dough with a ladle into the pan

4. Spread the banana pieces on the still moist dough, turn over after about 2 minutes and fry from the other side

12.7. Recipe for blueberry pancakes without sugar

Sunday morning and it should be something special? Then these sugar-free blueberry pancakes are perfect to start the day. The pancakes taste pure or with some maple syrup, honey or cream. Simply heavenly!

INGREDIENTS

- 110g of protein
- 50g cottage cheese
- 25g oatmeal
- 1 handful of blueberries
- 1 teaspoon vanilla flavor
- 0.5 teaspoon Stevia, liquid

PREPARATION

1. Pour all the ingredients (except the blueberries) into a mixing bowl and mix into a dough

2. Place half of the dough in a small pan and spread half of the blueberries on the still liquid dough

3. If the edge of the pancake bends slightly, turn the pancake to the other side and bake for another 3 minutes

4. Also proceed with the second half of the dough

Nutritional values

- Results: 2 Pancakes
- Calories: 196.7 kcal
- Fat: 4.1 g
- Carbohydrates: 16.7g
- Protein: 21.9g

12.8. Recipe for gluten-free blueberry buttermilk pancakes

For us the Sunday morning starts quite comfortably in the circle of the family with a lusciously laid breakfast table. Pancakes must not be missing - especially for the little ones. If you like something change on the table, should try the American version of the pancake. This is not only a bit thicker and fluffier than we are used to. Thanks to the buttermilk, these delicious blueberry pancakes also come loose and easy. Oh, and gluten-free and sugar-free, the pancakes are also natural!

Preparation time: 10 mins
Baking time: 15 minutes
Total time: 25 minutes

INGREDIENTS

- 225ml buttermilk
- 180g Flour, gluten free
- 160g blueberry
- 20g butter
- 1 grapefruit, juice
- 2 eggs
- 2 tsp baking powder, gluten-free
- 2 pinch of salt

PREPARATION

1. Place the flour, soda, baking powder, and salt in a bowl.

2. In a second bowl of buttermilk, juice of a grapefruit and eggs together and mix.

3. Now mix the contents of both mixing bowls and stir, leave to rest for 10 minutes

4. Heat some oil in a pan over medium heat.

5. Pour 3 tbsp. Of pancakes into the pan, add a few blueberries and bake for about 3 minutes, until the edge of the pancakes slightly arches.

6. Turn and bake from the other side. Finished.

Nutritional values

- Results: 7 Pancakes
- Calories: 100 kcal
- Fat: 2,5g
- Saturated Fatty Acids: 1.2g
- Carbohydrates: 16.1g
- Sugar: 0.8 g
- Iron: 0.7 g
- Protein: 2.8
- Cholesterol: 31mg

12.9. Recipe for a sugar free pannukaku

Pannukakku comes from the Finnish and is an incredibly delicious oven pancake. With a few raspberries and blueberries sprinkled, the pancake becomes a dessert, which is unparalleled. Attention! Danger of addiction.

Preparation time: 10 mins
Baking time: 15 minutes
Total time: 25 minutes

INGREDIENTS
- 150ml of milk
- Blueberries, raspberries
- 60g flour
- 1 egg
- 1.5 tsp Canderel
- 1 tsp butter, melted

- 1 pinch of salt
- Some vanilla flavor
- Some maple syrup

PREPARATION

1. Simply put all the ingredients (except the blueberries and raspberries) in a mixing bowl and mix to a creamy dough

2. Now spread an ovenproof form with baking paper or grease it with some butter and put in the dough

3. Sprinkle the raspberries and blueberries over it and let it go into the oven for about 15 minutes at 200 ° C

4. After the baking time has elapsed, briefly check with a shashlik spit whether the oven pancake is through

5. Allow to cool briefly, sprinkle with some maple syrup, then serve immediately

12.10. Recipe for apple and carrot muffins without sugar

Apple and carrot muffins along with walnuts and raisins are an absolutely heavenly creation! The raisins provide the necessary sweetness while the cinnamon and the walnuts give the muffins a Christmas flavor. But we can tell from our own experience that these muffins also taste in the high summer.

Preparation time: 10 mins
Baking time: 20 minutes
Total time: 30 minutes

INGREDIENTS

- 100ml buttermilk
- 100g apples
- 100g carrots
- 100g whole grain flour
- 40g raisins

- 20g walnuts, chopped
- 2.5 tbsp honey
- 1 teaspoon cinnamon
- 1 teaspoon Baking powder

PREPARATION

1. The apples and carrots fine grater

2. Add the remaining ingredients and mix well

3. Now spread the dough onto 8 muffin panes

4. At 180 degrees about 15 - 20 minutes in the oven

5. Then place the mold on a damp kitchen towel and let the whole thing cool down. Then release it from the mold

Nutritional values

- Returns: 6-8 pieces

- Calories: 754 kcal
- Fat: 24.7g
- Carbohydrates: 117.4g
- Protein: 10.5g

12.11. Recipe for apple full grain muffins without sugar

The whole grain is processed with all its valuable ingredients in the whole grain, while the edge layers as well as the seed which is valuable from a nutritional physiological point of view are removed. As a result, all the good dietary fibers and vital substances that are still contained in wholemeal flour are missing from the extract flour.A fact that definitely speaks for the use of whole grain flour. And these sugar-free apple full-grain muffins prove that one must definitely not make any taste cuts with wholemeal flour.

Preparation time: 20 minutes
Baking time: 25 minutes
Total time: 45 minutes

INGREDIENTS

- 400g apples
- 250ml of milk
- 150g whole grain flour
- 150g oatmeal
- 80g butter, melted
- 2 eggs
- 1 packet of baking soda
- 1 teaspoon cinnamon
- 1 pinch of salt
- Stevia

PREPARATION

1. Wash the apples, peel and cut into small cubes. Set aside

2. Stir the eggs with stevia, cinnamon, salt, milk and butter

3. Now add the flour and the baking powder with stirring

4.   Finally, remove the oat-meal and the apple pieces

5.   Put the dough into a baking dish and bake in a pre-heated oven at 200 ° C for about 25 to 30 minutes

Nutritional values

- Produces: 12 muffins
- Calories: 2151.6 kcal
- Fat: 102.3g
- Carbohydrates: 247.8g
- Protein: 45.0g

12.12. Recipe for banana muffins without sugar

Muffins is actually a pastry made from yeast dough from the UK, but it was brought to the United States by British immigrants in the 19th century and changed to what we know today as muffins.These delicious banana muffins please us mainly because they are without sugar and are also wonderfully loose-fluffy. This sugar-free recipe gives a total of 12 muffins.

Preparation time: 15 minutes
Baking time: 20 minutes
Total time: 35 minutes

INGREDIENTS

- 190g flour
- 80ml oil
- 4 bananas, ripe

- 2 eggs
- 2 hands full raisins
- 1 handful of walnuts, chopped
- 4 tbsp Canderel
- 2 tsp of baking soda
- 0.5 teaspoon of soda

PREPARATION

1. Stir the eggs with the oil

2. Grate the ripe bananas with a fork and add to the egg / oil mixture

3. Then add the flour, baking soda and soda and mix with a hand mixer

4. Then add the raisins and (if desired) the walnuts

5. Place the dough in the muffin mold, which is made with paper baking molds, and bake at 180 ° C for about 20 minutes until

the muffins have a golden-brown note.

Nutritional values

- Produces: 12 muffins
- Calories: 2396.8 kcal
- Fat: 123.0g
- Carbohydrates: 287.6g
- Protein: 22.9g

12.13. Recipe for blueberry without sugar

Blueberries (also called blueberries, black-berries or hayberries) belong to the family of heather plants. The blueberry is often also used as a healing plant. Thus the anthocyanins contained in blueberries are given an antioxidant and anti-inflammatory effect. Dried blueberries are used as an effective remedy for diarrhea due to pectins and tannins. Healing effect back and forth - these sugar-free blueberry suits are simply heavenly. So - let it taste you!

Preparation time:

Baking time: 20 minutes

Total time: 20 minutes

INGREDIENTS

- 270g Blueberries
- 250 g flour

- 175ml of milk
- 75g butter, soft
- 3 eggs
- 5 tablespoons maple syrup
- 2 tsp of baking soda
- 0.5 bottle Butter vanilla flavor

PREPARATION

1. Add the butter together with the milk, the eggs, the maple syrup and the aroma into a mixing bowl and mix with a hand mixer

2. Gradually add the flour and the baking powder to the dough and mix everything to a smooth dough

3. Now carefully place the blueberries under the dough

4. Place the dough into a baking dish, using 2 tablespoons

5. Now bake between 20 and 30 minutes in the circulating ether at 160 ° C

6. Towards the end of the baking time simply use a wooden stick to check whether the muffins are already finished (the muffins are ready when no dough sticks to the stick)

Nutritional values

- Calories: 1773.6 kcal
- Fat: 104.4g
- Carbohydrates: 171.4g
- Protein: 24.4g

12.14. Recipe for oat-blue muffins without sugar

Muffins - small cakes that are so diverse and delicious that we can not get enough of them. The mixture of blueberries and oat flakes gives the muffins a wonderfully strong flavor. Simply delicious!

Preparation time:

Baking time: 25 minutes

Total time: 25 minutes

INGREDIENTS

- 240g apple sauce
- 120g flour
- 100g blueberries
- 75g oatmeal, delicate
- 75 ml of milk
- 50g butter, melted
- 2 eggs

- 1 teaspoon cinnamon
- 1 teaspoon Baking powder
- 1 teaspoon of soda
- 1 teaspoon stevia powder
- 0.5 teaspoon salt

PREPARATION

1. Preheat the oven to 200 ° C

2. Put all ingredients (except the blueberries) in a bowl and mix to a smooth dough

3. Then remove the blueberries

4. Put the dough into a muffin mold and bake the muffins for about 25 minutes

Nutritional values

- Calories: 1623.3 kcal

- Fat: 75.5g
- Carbohydrates: 193.3g
- Protein: 31.4g

12.15. Recipe for an oatmeal raspberry chick

Oats are not among the healthiest and most nutritious grains. Even small amounts of nutrients supply our body with biotin as well as vitamin B1 and B6. Oatmeal for powerful fingernails, shining hair and a radiant complexion. In addition, oat flakes are very filling and have a positive effect on our digestion. The small fiber miracle we have processed here in a small, gluten- and sugar-free raspberry chickens to start healthy, sugar-free and saturated in the day.

Preparation time: 2 minutes
Baking time: 25 minutes
Total time: 27 minutes

INGREDIENTS
- 40ml almond milk
- 35g oatmeal

- 2 protein
- 1 handful of raspberries
- 2-3 tablespoons of coarse sugar
- 1 teaspoon Baking powder
- 1 teaspoon cinnamon
- 1 pinch of salt

PREPARATION

1. All ingredients except the raspberries in a bowl and stir

2. Now take the raspberries

3. Place the dough in a small ovenproof bowl

4. Now bake for 25 to 30 minutes at 180 ° C in the oven

5. Alternatively, add to the microwave for 3 minutes until the core of the cucumber is no longer liquid

6. Decorate with a few raspberries and still enjoy warm

Nutritional values

- Output: 1 person
- Serving size: Per ketch
- Calories: 265 kcal
- Fat: 5g
- Carbohydrates: 38g
- Sugar: 4g
- Iron: 9g
- Protein: 20g

12.16. Recipe for chocolate scones without sugar

Scones - who has ever been to the British Isles knows that the English like to enjoy this pastry for the traditional tea time. Right! Because the little pastries have it really in itself. In the following we would like to introduce you to a wonderfully chocolate-like version, which is not only gluten-free and low-carb, but - as it should be otherwise - naturally free from sugars. The taste does not break, we can promise you!

Preparation time: 20 minutes
Baking time: 15 minutes
Total time: 35 minutes

INGREDIENTS

- 240g almond flour
- 120ml milk

- 120g Chocolate Chips, sugar free
- 40g butter, soft
- 2 eggs
- 2 tablespoons of birch
- 1 teaspoon Baking powder
- 1 pinch of salt
- Coaster, dark, sugar free

PREPARATION

1. Preheat the oven to 160 ° C

2. Put the almond flour, the baking powder, the salt and the raw sugar into a bowl and mix the ingredients

3. Now add the butter, the eggs and the milk, and stir everything to a smooth dough

4. The Chocolate Chips

5. Form the dough into a ball and flatten it on a well-grounded

surface so that the dough is about 2 cm high

6. Now cut with a knife into eight equal-sized triangles and slightly offset on the baking sheet

7. Bake at 180 ° C for about 15 to 20 minutes until the scones have a slightly brownish color

8. After the scones are chilled, cover the scones. Finished

Nutritional values

- Portion Size: Pro Scone
- Calories: 171 kcal
- Fat: 14g
- Carbohydrates: 11g
- Iron: 2g
- Protein: 4g

12.17. Recipe for a sugar-free apple oatmeal slurry

If you are in a hurry in the morning and you're looking for a delicious, sugar-free breakfast that will make you start into the day, this apple oatmeal porridge is just right for you. The combination of apple, cinnamon and walnuts is a classic that tastes great. The creamy nutty note of the almond milk gives the apple porridge the finishing touch.

Preparation time: 15 minutes
Baking time:
Total time: 15 minutes

INGREDIENTS
- 8 tbsp almond milk, unsweetened
- 4 tbsp oatmeal, tender
- 0.5 apple, small grated

- 0,5 Banana, ripe
- 2-3 walnuts
- 1 teaspoon cinnamon
- Chia or linseed

PREPARATION

1. Put the oatmeal together with the almond milk and simmer the whole thing on a small flame until the oatmeal has slightly soaked the almond milk

2. Drill the apple and crush the banana

3. Place the oatmeal in a bowl and stir in the banana-apple mixture

4. Now add some walnut pieces and a few lei and chia seeds. Finished

5. If the sweetness of the fruit is not sufficient, the mash can be re-

fined with some honey or maple syrup

NUTRITIONAL VALUES

- Output: 1 person
- Calories: 169.8 kcal
- Fat: 5.8g
- Carbohydrates: 22.8g
- Protein: 5.3g

12.18. Crispy apple muesli without sugar

Crispy apple muesli with almond milk, just fresh from the oven and still sugar-free. Sounds too good to be true? Here is our recipe:

INGREDIENTS

- 1 apple
- 100ml of water
- 40ml almond milk
- 30g nuts, chopped
- 2 tsp cinnamon
- 1 teaspoon ginger
- ½ tsp

For the crumble:

- 40g oatmeal
- 1 tbsp butter, soft
- ½ tsp Rice syrup

PREPARATION

1. Preheat the oven to 180 ° C.

2. Put the water and the almond milk together with the spices cinnamon, ginger and nutmeg in a pan and simmer lightly.

3. Now peel the apple, cut into small pieces and add to the almond milk in the pot, until the apple pieces are beautifully soft.

4. In the meantime mix the ingredients for the crumble

5. Now place the apple in an oven-proof vessel, place the oatmeal crumble and the nuts over it and bake for 10 minutes in an oven golden brown.

6.   Just before serving, add some almond milk over the apple muesli. Best still warm to enjoy.

12.19. Recipe for a Chia-raspberry yoghurt without sugar

The mix of chia pudding, yogurt and raspberry puree is absolutely brilliant, I think! The Chia-raspberry yogurt is not difficult in the stomach, tastes fresh and fruity and is super-prepared, so that you have on the road or in the office something healthy fast. For me its the ideal snack - in the morning for breakfast, as a healthy dessert or for the small hunger between.

Preparation time: 5 minutes

Baking time:

Total time: 5 minutes

INGREDIENTS

- 100ml of milk
- 100g raspberries
- 100g yoghurt

- 2 tablespoons Chia seeds
- Honey as required

PREPARATION

1. Chia seeds together with the milk in a bowl and cold for several hours, stirring occasionally, so that no lumps form

2. Raspberries puree

3. Mix the yoghurt with a little honey

4. Then pour the yoghurt, chia pudding and raspberries into a glass jar and enjoy

Nutritional values

- Serving Size: Per serving
- Calories: 301 kcal
- Fat: 12.3g
- Carbohydrates: 30.5g
- Protein: 14g

12.20. Recipe for Chia Overnight Oats with Mango

If you have no desire and / or time to prepare a breakfast in the morning (or if you need a breakfast that can be well done), you should try this recipe. For the Overnight Oats one prepares - as the name suggests easily - on the evening before. Simply soak the oatmeal over night, add a few chia seeds and some fruit pulp, and you already have a wonderfully healthy breakfast that can be refined according to your mood - for example with cinnamon, nutmeg, vanilla or cocoa.

Preparation time: 10 mins
Baking time:
Total time: 10 mins

INGREDIENTS

- 100g natural yoghurt
- 100ml + 50ml almond milk
- 3 tablespoons oatmeal
- 2 tablespoons Chia seeds
- 1 mango

PREPARATION

1. Mix the chia seeds with 100ml almond milk and let them soak for about 30 minutes. Occasionally stir, so that the chia seeds do not lump.

2. Finely mash the oatmeal. Then add natural yogurt and 50ml of milk, set aside

3. Mango to a creamy fruit purée.

4. Then place the chia seed, the fruit and the oatmeal in a glass

and refrigerate overnight in the refrigerator

12.21. Recipe for a fitness muesli without sugar

Do you want to start healthy and easy in the morning, without the feeling that the breakfast is hard on the stomach? Then this fitness muesli without sugar is just right for you! The beauty of this muesli is that you always have the appropriate ingredients at home and it can be prepared so quickly and easily.

Possible variations of the fitness muesli are also:

- sesame
- Chopped almonds
- Saami mix
- Sunflower seeds
- Fruit by season

INGREDIENTS

- 300g natural yoghurt
- 50g oatmeal
- 2 hands full of walnuts
- 1 apple
- 1 banana
- 2 tsp honey

PREPARATION

1. Grate the apple finely and cut the banana into thin slices

2. Now add the remaining ingredients to the fruit and mix well

3. Serve with honey or stevia. Finished!

12.22. Recipe for an Almond Blueberry Chia Pudding

The beauty of chia pudding is that it is so diverse. Whether with cinnamon, with matcha or just with blueberries and almonds - who likes chia pudding, can free his creativity. And it will be healthy and delicious!

Preparation time: 10 mins
Baking time:
Total time: 10 mins

INGREDIENTS

- 150ml almond milk
- 80g blueberry, TK or fresh
- 2 tablespoons Chia seeds
- 2 tsp honey, optional
- 8-10 almonds, roughly chopped

PREPARATION

1. Chia seeds, blueberries, almond milk and honey, stir briefly and stir in the fridge for at least one or two hours (preferably overnight), stirring occasionally, so that the pudding does not clump

2. Before eating the almonds roughly chop and spread with a few blueberries on the pudding

12.23. Recipe for a Matcha Chia Pudding

Matcha is now also mutated in Germany to a trend drink, so much is certain. The green tea, which is ground to the finest powder, actually originates from Japanese cuisine and is not only served as a tea, but also as an ingredient for ice cream, chocolate or milk drinks. We have conjured here with the Matcha powder and a few Chia seeds a really delicious pudding. Really recommendable if you want to start healthy and easy in the morning.

Please note: Matcha is very stimulating. Therefore this pudding is not for children! Anyone who fights with sleep disorders or is sensitive to caffeine should also avoid it

Preparation time: 10 mins
Baking time:
Total time: 10 mins

INGREDIENTS

- 150ml almond milk
- 3 tbsp Chia seeds
- 2 tsp honey
- 0.5 teaspoon of Matcha tea
- 1 pinch of salt

PREPARATION

1. Almond milk, honey, salt and matcha

2. Now place the chia seeds in a bowl and place the milk-matcha mixture over it, stir well, so that the chia seeds are covered by the milk, put in the refrigerator and re-mix after 10 minutes, so that the Chia-Seeds do not lump

3. Ideally over night, otherwise 3-5 hours in the refrigerator cool, so that the Chia seeds can swell

12.24. Recipes for muesli without sugar

A full-fledged muesli is the ideal start to the day in many ways. But beware: the muesli, which are available in the supermarket, usually have an enormous sugar content. A sugar content of 40% is no exception. Therefore, you should ideally arrange your own muesli. There are no limits to the imagination.

Here are some suggestions for a self-assorted, full-fledged and sugar-free muesli:

- oatmeal
- Cereal flakes
- Amaranth, popped
- Buckwheat
- Spelled flakes
- Oatmeal flakes
- Brown millet

- Wheat germ flakes
- oats

NUTS AND SEEDS

- Chopped almonds
- Cashew Break
- Tigernuts
- Chopped pistachios
- sesame
- Pumpkin seeds
- Sunflower seeds
- Chia seeds
- linseed
- Hemp seed

SEASONAL FRUIT

- Small cut banana
- Grated apple
- Dried figs or dates
- Raisins

FURTHER INGREDIENTS

- Natural yoghurt
- milk
- Quark

The milk or the yogurt provide the morning protein boost. Protein is enormously important for our muscle and nerve tissue. And the complex carbohydrates ensure that our blood glucose levels rise slowly and we are therefore saturated until lunch, as well as being able to concentrate and concentrate. All of this naturally sugar-free, therefore also ideal for children as a start to the day.

12.25. Recipe for a sugar-free oatmeal mango muesli

This oatmeal mango tastes so good, because it can be prepared well, ultimately saturates and because you can take it well and thus can spoon easily on the way to work or at the desk. So you can start into the new day.

PS: I also liked a variation of cinnamon and apple! Or the mixture of banana cocoa powder ... or vanilla raspberry ... the muesli can be completely modified with some small variations

Preparation time: 10 mins
Baking time:
Total time: 10 min

INGREDIENTS

- 3 tbsp oatmeal, tender
- 0.5 mango
- 50g of milk
- 40g yogurt
- 2 tsp linseed
- Honey as required

PREPARATION

1. Add all the ingredients except for the mango to a closable vessel and mix well

2. Now the mango pieces to the muesli. Stir briefly

3. Close the container and place in the refrigerator overnight

4. The muesli tastes best when chilled and stays for up to 2 days

Nutritional values

- Output: 1 person
- Calories: 151.9 kcal
- Fat: 1.0g
- Carbohydrates: 30.1g
- Protein: 4.7 g

12.26. Recipe for a quinoa breakfast porridge

If you are fed up with muesli, bread or bread rolls and want to bring some change to breakfast in the morning, you should try this delicious quinoa breakfast. With pre-cooked quinoa, the mash is finished within a few minutes and saturates - at least that was the case with me - for several hours. Thumbs up for this super simple and super tasty quinoa breakfast slime.

INGREDIENTS

- 170ml almond milk
- 40g quinoa, pre-cooked
- 1 banana, ripe
- 1 pinch of cinnamon as needed

PREPARATION

1. Quinoa with hot water and put together with the almond milk into a cooking pot

2. Bring to a boil, then remove from the heat

3. Sprinkle the ripe banana with a fork and add to quino peppers

4. Mix well, sprinkle with a little cinnamon as needed and serve lukewarm

12.27. Recipe for an Overnight Chocolate Chia Pudding

If you want to start the day sweet and chocolaty in the day, the overnight chocolate-chia pudding should have found your favorite breakfast. Simply prepare on the eve, put in the refrigerator overnight and enjoy breakfast in the morning. Healthy, tasty, easy! We are just thrilled! You too?

Preparation time: 15 minutes
Baking time:
Total time: 15 minutes

INGREDIENTS

- 360 ml almond milk, unsweetened
- 60g Chia seeds

- 25g Cocoa powder, deoiled, un-sweetened
- 30 ml maple syrup
- 0.5 teaspoon cinnamon
- 0.25 teaspoon sea salt

PREPARATION

1. Combine all ingredients except the maple syrup in a bowl (or a blender) and mix well

2. As required with maple syrup sweet

3. Then place in the refrigerator for a few hours (typically overnight)

Nutritional values

- Results: 4 servings
- Serving Size: Per serving
- Calories: 133 kcal

- Fat: 8g
- Saturated Fatty Acids: 1.2g
- Carbohydrates: 17g
- Sugar: 9g
- Protein: 5.3g

12.28. Recipe for a Cinnamon Chia Pudding

The combination of Chia seeds and cinnamon is simply divine. For us, cinnamon can actually go pure into the yogurt, into the coffee (yes, really - tastes excellent!), Into the muesli and of course - how could it be different - into the Chia pudding. Just try it out! But beware - addiction!

INGREDIENTS

- 150ml almond milk
- 3 tbsp Chia seeds
- 1 teaspoon cinnamon
- 1 teaspoon agave juice, optional

PREPARATION

1. Put all ingredients in a bowl, stir well

2.   Stir again after about 10 minutes to ensure that the Chia seeds do not lump

3.   Now about 3 hours, preferably overnight in the refrigerator

4.   Before eating, sprinkle with some cinnamon

12.29. Recipe for cinnamon muesli without sugar

Sugar-free cinnamon crunchy sounds too good to be true? Just try our sugar-free muesli and we promise you - you will be thrilled. Here is our recipe:

Preparation time: 20 minutes
Baking time: 60 minutes
Total time: 1 hour 20 minutes

INGREDIENTS

- 320g oatmeal
- 100g almonds, donated
- 80g Pumpkin seeds
- 80g sunflower seeds
- 50g Flaxseed
- 50g raisins
- 6 tbsp apple sauce, sugar free
- 6 tbsp honey

- 4 tbsp Canderel
- 3 tablespoons sesame oil
- 2 tsp cinnamon
- 3 pinch of salt

PREPARATION

1. Preheat oven to 150 ° C

2. Add the oatmeal, the almonds, pumpkin and sunflower seeds, the linseed and the salt into a bowl. Put aside

3. Add the oil, 4 tbsp of canderel and 4 tbsp of apple sauce to a microwave-capable dish, heat for about 20 seconds in the microwave, stir and then add 4 tbsp of honey

4. Now add the honey paste over the dry ingredients, mix well so that the oatmeal and almonds are well-wetted

5. Then spread the crispbread uniformly on a baking tray with baking paper and bake for about 30 minutes in an oven

6. Add the remaining 2 tbsp celery and the remaining 2 tbsp.

7. After 30 minutes, remove the muesli from the oven and add the apple and honey mixture over the oatmeal

8. Now place it in the oven again and bake another 30 to 35 minutes crispy golden brown

9. Allow to cool completely, break into equally large pieces, mix with the raisins and fill in a airtight box

10. The muesli is enough for about 15 servings.

Nutritional values

- Returns: 15-20
- Serving Size: Total
- Calories: 3737.5 kcal
- Grease: 197.0g
- Carbohydrates: 349.0g
- Protein: 114.6g

12.30. Recipe for an apple-avocado fruit salad

The avocado bursts with precious minerals and trace elements as well as monounsaturated fatty acids. Together with walnuts and an apple, a deliciously healthy breakfast is served, which we would definitely recommend.

Preparation time: 15 minutes
Baking time:
Total time: 15 minutes

INGREDIENTS

- 1 avocado
- 1 apple
- 1 tbsp raisins
- 1 tbsp walnuts, chopped
- 0.5 tbsp honey
- 1 teaspoon lemon juice
- 2 pinch cinnamon

- 1 teaspoon water

PREPARATION

1.Peel the apple and cut into bite-size pieces

2.Together with 1 tsp water into a micro-wave-proof vessel and heat for one minute. Let cool down

3.Now mix the honey, lemon juice and cinnamon, if necessary with a little water to a dressing

4.Remove the avocado from the core, cut into bite size pieces and mix with the apple pieces

5.Add the dressing, stir well and finish with raisins and walnuts

12.31. Recipe for an avocado citrus salad with buttermilk dressing

This avocado-citrus salad is admittedly somewhat more elaborate in the preparation, but the result compensates in no time. The crunchy leaf salad, together with the lemony note, the buttermilk dressing and the crunchy croutons, create a taste experience that is unparalleled.

INGREDIENTS

- 100g leaf salad
- 1 avocado
- 1 orange
- 3-4 tablespoons of raspberries
- 50ml buttermilk
- 2 tsp lemon juice
- 1 tablespoon Greek yogurt
- 3 tsp of birch sugar

- 1 pinch of pepper
- 1 pinch of salt
- 4 tablespoons oatmeal
- 2 tablespoons sunflower seeds
- 2 tbsp almonds, donated
- 2 tablespoons of maple syrup
- 2 tablespoons sunflower oil
- 1 pinch of salt

PREPARATION

1. Wash the lettuce and cut into bite-size pieces together with the avocado, on two plates

2. fillet the Orange , add to the salad together with the raspberries, add a pinch of salt and a little pepper

Now go to the croutons :

3. Add oatmeal, sunflower seeds, almonds and salt to a bowl and mix well

4. Add sunflower oil and maple syrup

5. Then spread on a baking sheet laid out with baking paper and bake crisply at 180 ° C for about 15 to 20 minutes (mix occasionally, so that the croutons are golden brown on all sides)

6. After the baking time has elapsed, let it cool completely and then break into small pieces

7. Buttermilk dressing:

8. Combine all the ingredients for the dressing and mix with a magic wand or snow bean

9. Bring over the salad and sprinkle over the croutons

12.32. Recipe for a Banana Chocolate Smoothie Bowl

Admittedly, the combination of banana and chocolate is a classic and is quite popular. This was shown once again in the preparation of this delightfully delicious, sugar-free Smoothie Bowl.

Suitable as topping are:

- Chia seeds
- sesame
- Coconut flakes
- Planed almonds

Preparation time: 15 minutes
Baking time:
Total time: 15 minutes

INGREDIENTS

- 250g Soy Yoghurt

- 1 banana
- 1 tablespoon cocoa powder
- Toppings as required

PREPARATION

Place the soy yoghurt together with the banana and the cocoa powder in a blender or alternatively mix with a blender. Fill in a bowl. Now decorate with the topping at will.

Nutritional values

- Output: 1 person
- Serving Size: Per serving
- Calories: 260.2 kcal
- Fat: 6.1 g
- Carbohydrates: 39.5g
- Protein: 10.0g

12.33. Recipe for a Blueberry breakfast salad

Have we ever mentioned that we are absolutely fans of breakfast salads? Probably already. Since breakfast salads are still completely unknown, you can not mention that often enough. Because the small, healthy vitamin bombs are an ideal opportunity for those who want to start the day sweet, but also healthy and nutritious. The combination of green, crunchy lettuce leaves, nuts and fruits is convincing not only from a nutritional point of view, but also from a taste point of view.

Preparation time: 25 minutes
Baking time:
Total time: 25 minutes

INGREDIENTS

- 2 Romana lettuce
- 300g blueberries
- 2 oranges
- 100ml rapeseed oil
- 10 Walnuts, chopped
- 2 tablespoons of birch
- 1 pinch of salt

PREPARATION

1. Chop the lettuce, dry and spin on 2 plates

2. Oranges and add to the salad together with half of the blueberries

3. Now we come to the dressing: the second half of the blueberries mix well with rapeseed oil, Xylitol and salt and give over the salad

4. Sprinkle with the walnuts and serve immediately

Nutritional values

- It can accommodate up to 2 people
- Serving Size: Per serving
- Calories: 746.5g
- Fat: 64.4g
- Carbohydrates: 26.7g
- Protein: 8,4g

12.34. Recipe for a blueberry quinoa bowl without sugar

Life can be so easy! Three ingredients, more does not need to start the day with a smile. Because with this Blaubeer-Quinoa-Bowl you are guaranteed a lot of good. Quinoa is full of healthy protein and is bursting with mineral and fiber. The blueberries are small but fine vitamin bombs, which strengthen the immune system and - one hears and astonishes - by the anthocyanins of the premature skin aging contained in them. So the morning can begin.

Preparation time:
Baking time: 20 minutes
Total time: 20 minutes

INGREDIENTS

- 450ml almond milk
- 200g blueberry
- 150 g of quinoa, cooled
- 1 tablespoon agave juice, as desired

PREPARATION

1. Wash Quinoa under running water. Then bring to a boil in a pot with the almond milk. Then reduce heat and let simmer for about 20 minutes.

2. Stir in the blueberries and add Agave Juice as desired.

3. Serve immediately - lukewarm tastes best!

12.35. Recipe for a Chai Smoothie Bowl Without Sugar

In Southeast Asia, Chai Tee is the mixture of black tea, milk and various spices like cinnamon, cardamom, cloves, nutmeg, Indian bay leaves and pepper. However, Chai tea can not only drink. Here I show you how you can prepare a warming and delightfully smooth Smoothie Bowl from the spice tea. So the chai tea is now spooned!

Preparation time: 15 minutes
Baking time:
Total time: 15 minutes

INGREDIENTS

- 150ml Chai tea, cold
- 4 tablespoons soy yoghurt
- 3 tablespoons oat bran flakes

- 1 banana, ripe
- 1 date
- 10 almonds
- 1 teaspoon Chia seeds
- 1 teaspoon cinnamon
- 0.5 teaspoon of nutmeg
- 1 pinch ginger, ground

PREPARATION

1.Add the chai tea, yogurt, oat bran, date, half a banana, nutmeg and cinnamon to a blender, pour well, leave to stand for about 10 minutes (so that the oat bran flakes can have an ideal consistency)

2.With almonds, the other half of the banana and chia seeds decorate - finished!

12.36. Recipe for an oatmeal quinoa salad

Oatmeal, millet, quinoa and blueberries are the main ingredients of this delicious muesli. Prepared the evening before, the muesli is a perfect breakfast for all those who want to start their day in the morning, but have little time.

Preparation time: 70 minutes
Baking time: 20 minutes
Total time: 1 hour 30 minutes

INGREDIENTS

- 250g Soy Yoghurt
- 30g of nuts
- 3 tablespoons of blueberries
- 2 tablespoons oatmeal
- 2 tbsp quinoa
- 2 tablespoons of millet
- 2 tsp oil

- 2 pinch of salt
- 0.5 lemon (zest and juice)
- water
- Maple syrup as desired

PREPARATION

1. Place quinoa and millet in a sieve and rinse with hot water for about one minute. Drain well

2. Add oatmeal and set aside

3. Heat the oil in a frying pan, add the oatmeal mix to the pan for 2-3 minutes and lightly fry while stirring constantly

4. Ml of water, the salt and halves of half a lemon into a cooking pot and bring to a boil

5. Reduce heat and simmer for about 20 minutes

6. Remove from heat and allow to cool for at least 30 minutes. Now add the remaining citron tarts

7. Maple syrup, yoghurt, 1 teaspoon olive oil and lemon juice into a large bowl and mix well

8. While the nuts are roasting in a pan (without oil)

9. Now add the nuts together with the blueberries and the dressing over the oatmeal mix and let them pull in the fridge overnight

12.37. Recipe for a vegan breakfast salad

A vegan breakfast salad? Sounds strange, we must be right. But at the latest after you have tasted the first bite of this salad, you will be enthusiastic. Full of healthy vitamins and minerals, this breakfast salad can be prepared perfectly, making it perfect for on the go.

Preparation time: 20 minutes

Baking time:

Total time: 20 minutes

INGREDIENTS

- 2 hands full of baby spinach
- 1 banana
- 1 orange
- 0.5 apple
- 4 strawberries
- 1 handful of walnuts

- 2 tablespoons of lemon juice
- 1 tbsp of Chia seeds
- 1 tbsp honey

PREPARATION

1. Wash the spinach and cut into bite-size pieces, place on a plate. Then wash the fruit and cut it in small pieces, decoratively on the spinach.

2. Mix the dressing from lemon juice, honey and chia seeds and pour over the salad.

Nutritional values

- Output: 1 person
- Calories: 345.3 kcal
- Fat: 7.1 g
- Carbohydrates: 63.4g
- Protein: 4.7 g

12.38. Quinoa fruit salad with honey and lime dressing

The title of the recipe suggests an extraordinary taste experience, so much is certain. And we can tell you for sure that this recipe has it in itself. So we do not talk long for the hot mash and instead go directly to the cooking spoon!

Preparation time: 20 minutes
Baking time:
Total time: 20 minutes

INGREDIENTS

- 300g mango, diced
- 300ml of water
- 170g quinoa
- 160g strawberries, diced
- 150g blueberry
- 1 pinch of salt

- 1 lime, juice

- 3 tbsp honey

- 2 tablespoons mint leaves, finely chopped

PREPARATION

1. Put quinoa, water and salt in a saucepan and bring to a boil

2. Cook for about 5 minutes, then reduce the temperature to medium heat and simmer for an additional 15 minutes

3. Now allow Quinoa to cool to room temperature

4. You can already prepare the dressing. Add the lime juice, the honey and the finely-cut mint and mix well

5. Now add quinoa, fruit and dressing, mix well and spread in bowls

13. Recipes for babies without sugar

The fact that babies should not come into contact with sugar and sugar has nothing to do at all in baby food, should be understood by itself. When choosing baby foods, the first baby biscuits or the first birthday cake, we make a decision as a parent. Are we leading our children to the low consumption of sugar or are we trying to make it sugar free? I know I can not keep my children away from sugar forever. I do not want that at all. What I want is to give them a good and healthy start into life and to teach them a conscious handling of sugar. I think that the taste buds can quickly deaden and that one does not have to spoil his children with sweet. Rather, I would like to spoil them in a different way. With attention and love. Sugar has nothing to look for.

When should I start with the introduction of complementary foods?

Between the 4th and 6th month. Before the 17th week of life the baby's bowel is not yet ready for breeding. Pre milk or mother's milk is the order of the day.

If the introduction of complementary food is pending, you should give the first spoonful of porridge in a day where no appointments are required and you have enough time to try the first attempts with peace and patience. Since the feeding at the beginning in the kitchen can cause a lot of chaos and the first spoon mash mostly not where they should be, one should start with the food as much as possible in a day, where you are half-happy and a little stressed.

In addition, it must be borne in mind that the babies are usually once overwhelmed with the food presented on the spoon. The mash is then pushed out once again with the tongue and after a few spoons the baby becomes impatient and again demands the bottle. So that the end of the food does not end at the end in a single shouting, you should give the first spoonful of bread usually between two meals. Because the little mouse has hungry, it becomes all the more difficult to convince her to take the porridge.

Even if you have a lot of patience at the beginning of the introduction of complementary food, and our twins sometimes refuse to eat more mushrooms after a few spoons, we have never compelled or forced them to continue eating. We believe its important, that they associate with the food something positive that the food is fun.

What ingredients should I use for the food?

The best is fresh organic food. We started with the classic. At midday, there was carrot in the first week, in week 2 I added potatoes and in week 3, turkeys added.

It is a good start to use sweet vegetables like carrots, parsnips or pumpkins. This is easily reminiscent of the sweet taste of the mother's milk and increases the chances that the baby's porridge is actually eaten. However, in the case of carrots and potatoes it must be remembered that they can quickly lead to constipation. Therefore, I advise to slow down and introduce a maximum of one vegetable per week.

From the 5th month the following ingredients can be tried:

vegetables	Carrots
	Potato

	Pumpkin
	Parsnips
	Sweet potato
	Courgette
meat	poultry
	lamb
	Cattle
	pig
Fruit (as mus or juice)	Apple
	avocado
	banana
	pear
	melon
cereals	semolina
	oatmeal
	Millet (flakes)
	Cornmeal
	Rice (flakes)

Others	Melt flakes
	Rapeseed oil

From the 7th month the following ingredients can be tried:

vegetables	Cauliflower
	Broccoli
	Fennel
	Kohlrabi
	celery root
	Asparagus
	Spinach
	Romanesco brocolli
	Tomatoes
meat	so
Fruit	apricot
	Orange
	mango
	peach

cereals	couscous
Others	Rapeseed oil

Food such as berries, kiwi, bread, noodles, fish or cheese are only available from the 9th month or later.

And which foods are taboo in the first year of life?

Some food should be dispensed with in the first year of life. This includes:

- Leaf Salad (cannot be chewed only by babies)

- Honey (honey can contain spores that mature in the infant's intestine, and in the worst case, this can lead to death)

- (Although they are healthy, have a partial but strongly inflated effect)

- Cheese (the high protein and mineral content stresses the kidneys too much)

- Cold-pressed oils (the pollutants contained therein can not be broken down by the baby's liver)

- Cow's milk, pure (the high protein content stresses the kidneys too much)

- Nuts (Attention: Danger of suffocation!)

- Quark (the high protein content stresses the kidneys too much)

- Raw eggs (salmonella risk)

- Cream (the high protein content stresses the kidneys too much)

- Salt (stresses the kidneys too much)

- Sharp spices (rarely tolerated)

- Sweeteners

Do I have to cook fresh every day?

There is a clear No to this question! I have always made it in the preparation of the mash so that I have boiled larger quantities, everything has been filled into ice cubes and then frozen. At least, this applies to the vegetable, fruit and meat sludge. I always had fresh potatoes, avocado and bananas.

Which baby's porridge cannot be frozen?

I always prepared fresh potatoes as the potato in the freezer not only changes its consistency and becomes watery after thawing, but because it also loses taste.

Avocados become bitter when frozen. Also melon and banana I always freshly mixed under the mash.

What does a food plan look like?

With the food is started between the 4th and 6th month.

The first meal to be served is the lunch meal. Thus the stomach has enough time to devote itself to the sleeping of the digestive system. We started in week 1 with carrot porridge. A teaspoonful of rapeseed oil is added to the carrot pulp so that the vitamins can be better absorbed by the body. In the second week came mashed potatoes and in the third week meat (turkey, beef, pork - best organic!). It was drunk between boiled water. You can also take tea, but we had little luck with our little ones. The two liked lukewarm water.

In order for a milk meal to be completely replaced, the end product should be about 200 grams, which is composed according to the Research Institute for Child Nutrition (FKE) as follows:

- 90-100g of vegetables

- 40-60g potatoes

- 30-45g fruit juice or fruit sauce

- 20-30g of meat

- 8-10g rapeseed oil

The next meal, which is converted, is the evening meal. Between the 6th and 8th month the milk-cereal is introduced. Instant porridge or semolina or milk sludge from the vial usually contain not a little sugar. We therefore always take rice or melt flakes with 100ml of whole milk and 100ml of water, let the whole boil up once. Here again, drinking should not be forgotten!

Finally, between the 7th and 9th month, the fruit-cereal mash is introduced which replaces a dairy meal either before or in the afternoon. From now on there are three times a day porridge plus one to two milk meals.

And what happens from the 10th month?

From the 10th month the small ones should slowly but surely be accustomed to solid food. So, the vegetable potato and pork is served at noon for a hot meal. I cook quite simply for my two mice the same as for us - but of course completely unseasoned - and cut it into small bites so that they can take their fingerfood as they please.

The evening milk and cereal bread goes into a bread meal and from the fruit-cereal two snacks in the morning and afternoon, which can for example consist of yoghurt, fruits or vegetables.

Recipes for babies from the 4th month:

- Recipe for an avocado apple gruel
- Recipe for a pumpkin cereal

Recipes for babies from the 10th month:

- Recipe for a baby cappuccino without sugar
- Recipe for baby biscuits without sugar
- Recipe for spelled whole corn without sugar
- Recipe for spelled waffles with maple syrup
- Recipe for vanilla without sugar
- Recipe for whole grain without sugar

13.1. Recipe for an avocado apple porridge without sugar

While carrots are often given to the start in the diet, other countries such as New Zealand often find avocados. The creamy consistency of the avocado, the unsaturated fatty acids and the amount of vital vitamins such as vitamin A, vitamin D, vitamin E, vitamin K, alpha carotene, beta carotene, lutein, lycopene and zeaxanthin make avocado a reasonably popular one Fruit for the baby porridge. Together with some applesauce, one can quickly conjured up a baby slime, which tasted so delicious. The avocado apple mash can be given from the fourth month.

INGREDIENTS

- 1 avocado

- 3 tbsp apple sauce, self-cooked, unmelted
- 1 tbsp water, boiled

PREPARATION

Pour the ingredients into a blender and finely puree

13.2. Recipe for a pumpkin cereal

The pumpkin is a classic autumn and winter vegetable. The gourd is suitable for baby food because it is not only low in fiber and therefore very easily digestible, but also very healthy, since the pumpkin is rich in mineral and nutrients as well as beta-carotene, iron and potassium. The pumpkin cereal can already be given as the first milk meal from the 4th month.

INGREDIENTS

- 125g Hokkaido pumpkin (the rest can be super frozen), alternatively 1 glass of pumpkin pure
- 50g of milk
- 50ml of water
- 3 tbsp of cereal (eg oat, meal)
- 1 teaspoon rapeseed oil

PREPARATION

1.   Boil milk and water, add pumpkin puree and rapeseed oil with stirring, and allow to cool to the desired temperature

13.3. Recipe for a baby cappuccino without sugar

Small children love to be with their parents. When I drink my morning cappuccino, there is a baby cappuccino for the little ones. The fact that a few vitamins are included, I find, of course, the better. Here comes the recipe ...

INGREDIENTS

- 150ml of milk
- 1 banana, ripe
- 10g oat bran

PREPARATION

1. Grate the banana with a fork
2. Add oat bran and 100ml of milk, puree and pour into a mug

3. Sprinkle the remaining milk and drizzle on the banana milk

Nutritional values

- Output: 1 person
- Serving Size: Per serving
- Calories: 171 kcal
- Grease: 3.0g
- Carbohydrates: 26.6g
- Sugar: 15.9g
  Protein: 7.4 g

13.4. Recipe for baby biscuits without sugar

Today many mothers and fathers are of the opinion that babies and toddlers should grow up without sugar.

In the certainty that the small ones can not be distant from sugar-containing foods anyway, they want at least to ensure that the baby and toddler's diet remains largely sugar-free. The following baby biscuits are suitable from the 11th month. They just come out with two ingredients and taste deliciously fruity. Here comes our recipe for sugar-free baby biscuits:

Preparation time: 5 minutes
Baking time: 15 minutes
Total time: 20 minutes

INGREDIENTS

- 200g apple sauce, sugar free
- 100g oatmeal

PREPARATION

1. Mix the two ingredients to form a sticky mass

2. Now take two teaspoons to the hand and place small dough mountains on a baking sheet laid out with baking paper

3. In the meantime, pre-heat the oven to 160 ° C

4. Now the dough mountains come in the oven for about 15 minutes. The baby's biscuits are ready.

13.5. Recipe for spelled biscuits without sugar

If you are traveling with small children, it is always helpful if you have something to nibble on hand. Because when it is time for shopping or the waiting time at the pediatrician pulls like gum, our sugar-free spelled biscuits are worth the gold. The little ones are busy for a while and you are more relaxed. The spelled biscuits are also suitable from the 11th month.

Preparation time: 15 minutes

Baking time: 15 minutes

Total time: 30 minutes

INGREDIENTS

- 200g spelled full grain flour
- 100g butter
- 1 banana, large, ripe

PREPARATION

1. Mix all the ingredients well and roll on a floured surface with a rolling pin.

2. Now stick out to your liking.

3. Preheat the oven to 200 degrees and bake the cookies for 15 minutes

13.6. Recipe for spelled waffles with maple syrup

Anyone who does not have to consume sugar and sugar, but can not leave his hands of freshly baked wafers, might have found a delicious alternative with these sugar-free spelled waffles. But of course, the spelled waffles are not just for adults. Because even babies from the 11th month of life may eat from the waffles.

Preparation time: 20 minutes
Baking time:
Total time: 20 minutes

INGREDIENTS
- 250g spelled full grain flour
- 250ml whole milk
- 125g butter, soft
- 2 eggs

- 1 teaspoon Baking powder
- Maple syrup as required

PREPARATION

1. Put all ingredients in a mixing bowl and mix well

2. Now bake the waffles portion wise in the waffle iron

13.7. Recipe for vanilla without sugar

Preparation time: 15 minutes

Baking time: 15 minutes

Total time: 30 minutes

INGREDIENTS

- 260g spelled flour
- 200g butter
- 100g pear juice
- 100g almonds, ground
- 2 Msp. Vanilla

PREPARATION

1. Combine all the ingredients into a crusty dough, place in the refrigerator for about 30 minutes.

2. Then shape from the dough uniformly large kipferl, on a baking sheet laid with baking sheet

and bake between 10 and 15 minutes in the pre-heated oven at 180 ° C light.

3. For the not completely sugar-free variant the still hot Vanilla kipferl if necessary still with some powdered sugar dust.

13.8. Recipe for baby whole grain without sugar

Some wholemeal flour, a little butter and two bananas - the world can be so simple! With just three ingredients and ten minutes of preparation, delicious, sugar-free wholemeal tarts are prepared in null commingles, which are suitable for babies from the age of 11 months.

Preparation time: 10 mins
Baking time: 15 minutes
Total time: 25 minutes

INGREDIENTS

- 200g whole grain flour
- 150g butter, soft
- 2 bananas, ripe

PREPARATION

1. Grate the bananas with a fork

2. Preheat the oven to 180 ° C

3. Put all ingredients in a mixing bowl and knead together

4. Roll the dough into small balls, place on a baking tray, bake flat and bake for 15 to 20 minutes.

5. Alternatively roll out the dough with a rolling pin and cut out the pastry biscuit.

Nutritional values

- Results: 50 full grain
- Serving Size: Pro Taler
- Calories: 22.2 kcal
- Fat: 2,5g
- Carbohydrates: 0.02g
- Sugar: 0.02g
- Protein: 0.02g

Other Books by the Author

10 Day Green Smoothies Cleanse
http://amzn.to/2lhYfB7

Lose Fat and Keep it Off Forever
http://amzn.to/2kKvZn7

http://amzn.to/2kKyTbr

http://amzn.to/2kT0PMS

Made in the USA
Middletown, DE
28 February 2017